SOCIAL POLICY & AGING

A Critical Perspective

DISCARDED

Carroll L. Estes
and Associates

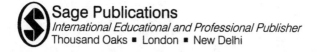

Sage Publications
International Educational and Professional Publisher
Thousand Oaks ▪ London ▪ New Delhi

Carroll L. Estes and Associates

Robert R. Alford

Elizabeth A. Binney

Julia E. Bradsher

Liz Close

Chiquita A. Collins

Anne Hays Egan

Charlene Harrington

Karen W. Linkins

Marty Lynch

Jane L. Mahakian

David N. Pellow

Steven P. Wallace

Tracy A. Weitz

For information:

Sage Publications, Inc.
2455 Teller Road
Thousand Oaks, California 91320
E-mail: order@sagepub.com

Sage Publications Ltd.
6 Bonhill Street
London EC2A 4PU
United Kingdom

Sage Publications India Pvt. Ltd.
M-32 Market
Greater Kailash I
New Delhi 110 048 India

Printed in the United States of America

Library of Congress Cataloging-in-Publication Data

Social policy and aging: A critical perspective / by Carroll L. Estes
and Associates.
   p. Cm.
Includes bibliographical references and index.
  ISBN 0-8039-7346-2 (cloth: acid-free paper) — ISBN 0-8039-7347-0
(pbk.: acid-free paper)
  1. Aged—United States. 2. Aging—United States. 3. Aged—Government
policy—United States. 4. Aged—Medical care—United States. 5. Social
stratification—United States. I. Carroll L. Estes and Associates.
  HQ1064.U5 S5945 2000
  305.26'0973—dc21   00-010918

     02   03   10   9   8   7   6   5   4   3   2

Acquiring Editor:	Jim Brace-Thompson
Editorial Assistant:	Anna Howland
Production Editor:	Diana E. Axelsen
Editorial Assistant:	Victoria Cheng
Copy Editor:	Linda Gray
Typesetter/Designer:	Denyse Dunn
Indexer:	Jeanne Busemeyer
Cover Designer:	Michelle Lee

Contents

Dedicated to

Maggie Kuhn
*mentor, friend, and visionary for social justice and
founder of the Gray Panthers*

Tish Sommers
*mentor, friend, and feminist guide and
founder of the Older Women's League*

Solomon Davis
*late student, colleague, and friend
whose life and example taught us the importance of this work*

Duskie Lynn Estes
and to the generations to follow:
The best reason for a critical perspective and praxis

Introduction

Carroll L. Estes

S ocial Policy and Aging: A Critical Perspective offers the only comprehensive book-length treatment of what is a new and widely recognized
theoretical paradigm and approach in social gerontology—the political
economy of aging. The book is authored by the scholar who is widely
acknowledged and credited as the founder and key thinker in the
political economy of aging in the United States and internationally
(Bengtson, Burgess, & Parrott, 1997; Bengtson & Schaie, 1999; Hendricks,
1992; Hendricks & Leedham, 1991; Marshall, 1996, 1999; Phillipson,
1998; Quadagno & Reid, 1999; Walker, 1999).

The body of work presented in this volume, in developing and theorizing this critical perspective, aims to contribute to the understanding
of old age and aging in the context of problems and issues of the larger
social order in the world's most advanced capitalist nation, the United
States of America. Since the first writing on the political economy of
aging in 1979 (Estes, 1979), there has been growing recognition and
now full incorporation of Estes's critical perspective as one of the
major paradigms in the field of aging.

In the past 20 years, there has been a revolution in the globalization
of capital and in health care restructuring as well as major theoretical advances in work on the welfare state and in social gerontological theory,
both of which are addressed in this new volume. Included in the book is
an exposition of theoretical developments and their application to the issue
of social policy and aging. The 11 chapters that compose this volume explore
the issue of social policy of aging from various components of the political economy model. They include overlapping and interwoven themes,
each taking a slightly different orientation or specific topic of analysis.

In Chapter 1, Estes proposes a theoretical multilevel analytical framework that advances her previous work on social constructionism and the political economy perspectives, refined and expanded by concepts drawn from critical perspectives, feminist theories, and cultural studies (see Table I.1). This framework examines the political, economic, and social conflicts at and between the institutional levels of postindustrial capital, the state, the sex/gender system, and the public/citizen and including the mesolevel of the medical-industrial complex and the aging enterprise. Conflicts over social policy are power struggles that must be analyzed in terms of reigning and competing ideologies and the "interlocking systems of oppression" of race, class, gender, and age to understand the social construction of aging and the aged and the formation of social policy.

In Chapter 2, Estes, Linkins, and Binney review critical perspectives on aging and health from gerontological, critical, political, feminist, and cultural foundations. The authors highlight specific critical perspectives that contribute to the analytical capabilities of the theoretical framework advanced in Chapter 1 and discuss the application of a critical theoretical approach to social policy and aging.

In Chapter 3, Estes, Wallace, Linkins, and Binney discuss four social processes that shape old age, aging, and policy formation: medicalization, commodification, privatization, and rationalization. The social construction of aging as a medical problem and the resulting production of medical commodities are analyzed in terms of the relations between postindustrial capital and the state. With the realization of profitability, the transition to privately dominated provision of commodified medical services formed the foundation for the medical-industrial complex and the aging enterprise. Attempts to rationalize this transformation have led to the restructuring of health care in pursuit of efficiency and cost reduction.

In Chapter 4, Estes, Alford, and Egan examine in greater detail the role played by the nonprofit sector in relation to postindustrial capital and the state. This chapter explores the literature on crisis and capitalism and crisis and the state to understand how the nonprofit health and social services sector may be employed both as a buffer and as a resource for capital and how the state responds to its own legitimation crisis tendencies. A detailed review of crisis theory precedes a critical analysis of the political economy of nonprofit service provision.

In Chapter 5, Estes documents the social construction of crisis and its political uses in the definition and treatment of "the problem" of

Table I.1 Development of the Estes Model of the Political Economy of Aging

Theories	Dates Introduced
Conflict	1972, 1976
Organizational	1972, 1976
Sociology of knowledge	1972, 1976
Symbolic interaction (social constructionism and labeling)	1972, 1976, 1980
Political economy	1979
Feminist	1984
Critical	1991
Cultural studies	1999

SOURCES: Estes (1972, 1976, 1979, 1980, 1991, 1999b) and Estes, Gerard, and Clarke (1984).

the aged and the framing of social policy options as exemplified by the debate over the privatization of Social Security. The chapter uses multiple levels of the theoretical framework described in Chapter 1 to analyze the roles of postindustrial capital, the state, and ideology, with particular attention to the media.

In Chapter 6, Estes proposes a framework to understand the political economy of gender and aging that identifies aging as both a gender and a women's issue. This chapter analyzes the particular situation of older women within the gendered state and women's roles in social institutions and social policy. The state, in conflicts over capital and resources, promotes and reproduces the dominant institutions that support the sex/gender system and that create and perpetuate the economic and social dependency of women.

In Chapter 7, Collins, Estes, and Bradsher investigate the issue of dependency and its social construction in greater detail. The inequality that results from dependency is analyzed across the dimensions of the interlocking systems of oppression: class, gender, and race/ethnicity, with age providing another dimension of analysis to this perspective. Economic and social well-being are examined, in conjunction with social support, mortality, morbidity, and the use of health care.

In Chapter 8, Estes, Harrington, and Pellow review in detail the establishment of the medical-industrial complex and the aging enterprise, which taken together, represent a key mesolevel of analysis in the theoretical framework introduced in Chapter 1. The structure of the health care industry is examined in light of the role of capital (i.e., the market) and the state. This chapter describes changes in the medical care industry, growth and consolidation, horizontal and vertical integration, diversification and globalization, and the need for regulation.

In Chapter 9, Estes, Mahakian, and Weitz provide a critique of the construction of the concepts of successful and "productive" aging. With the recognition of the social determinants of health and aging, social policy has attempted to frame the issue of aging in positive ways to improve health conditions and outcomes for the elderly. The authors contend that the promotion of productive aging, although well-intentioned, perpetuates the construction of aging as an individual problem rather than a sociocultural one and continues to prioritize the interests of capital and the state over the existing needs of the aged. Productive aging ignores and perpetuates the inequalities represented in the interlocking systems of oppression.

In Chapter 10, Lynch and Estes locate the underdevelopment of community-based long-term care within a larger political and economic context. This chapter examines the economic, political, and sociocultural factors that have influenced the development of long-term care systems in the United States and mapped the future directions of policy and service. With the demographic changes of the 21st century, the issues related to long-term care are of paramount importance.

In Chapter 11, Close, Estes, and Linkins address the political economy of health work, analyzing the systemic characteristics of the labor involved in the provision of health, social, and long-term care services. This chapter examines health work in the capitalist economy, the informalization of health work, and the policy environment in which health work is situated. The authors delineate the political and economic assumptions made about the nature (and the costs) of health work that undergird social policy of aging in a capitalist society.

Estes concludes this volume with observations on social policy, theory, and research. These concluding remarks summarize and contextualize the most salient issues raised in the book and direct attention to the future of empirical and theoretical work in the field of social policy and aging.

Acknowledgments

There are many individuals to whom we owe a debt of gratitude for their part in making this book possible. We want to acknowledge that this volume builds on earlier work with our colleagues, Lenore Gerard, James Swan, and Jane Sprague Zones, with whom *Political Economy, Health, and Aging* was written in 1984. Ted Benjamin, Charlene Harrington, Robert Newcomer, Jim Swan, and Juanita Wood contributed insights in the early years as policy research colleagues. Ideas further developed and elaborated here have appeared in the three volumes of books coedited with colleague and friend, Meredith Minkler *(Readings in the Political Economy of Aging,* 1984; *Critical Perspectives on Aging,* 1991; and *Critical Gerontology,* 1999).

Encyclopedic knowledge of Medicare, Social Security, and health statistics has been generously offered by Robert Ball, Shirley Chater, Philip Lee, and Dorothy Rice. Their insights and experience in the nation's capitol as two U.S. Commissioners of Social Security, the Assistant Secretary for Health, U.S. Department of Health and Human Services, and Director of the National Center for Health Statistics, respectively, have illuminated the historical context and policy considerations undergirding the issues covered in the book. Karen Davis, President of the Commonwealth Fund, has been an important mentor on the research, policy, and professional level.

Five individuals have been especially influential as intellectual mentors and advisers in developing the theoretical underpinnings of the framework used here: Randall Collins, Joseph Gusfield, James O'Connor, and the late Herbert Blumer and Alvin Gouldner. Fred Koenig and John Walton, early teachers and mentors, opened us to the value of a critical perspective. Colleagues and scholars in gerontology and in feminist studies whose writing, discussions, and critiques have advanced our thinking include Robert Binstock, Timothy Diamond, Lou Glasse, Vida Jones, Madonna Harrington Meyer, Jon Hendricks, Vic Marshall, Rick Moody, Marilyn Moon, John Myles, Anabel Pelham, Jill Quadagno, John Rother, Tim Smeeding, and Josh Wiener in the United States and Canada; Chris Phillipson, Anne Showstack Sassoon, and Alan Walker in the United Kingdom; Anne Marie Guillemard in France; and Anna Howe in Australia. Jonathon Showstack deepened our understanding of health policy and health services, and Deb Briceland-Betts expanded our understanding of older women's issues.

Many funders have supported parts of the research and conceptual development contained herein: the Administration on Aging (AoA), Department of Health and Human Services (DHHS), the AARP/Andrus Foundation, the Agency for Health Care Policy and Research (AHCPR), the Aspen Institute Nonprofit Sector Research Fund, the Frost Foundation, the DHHS Health Care Financing Administration (HCFA), the Kaiser Family Foundation, the Meyer Charitable Trusts, the Pew Charitable Trusts, the Public Welfare Foundation, the Retirement Research Foundation, the Robert Wood Johnson Foundation, and the DHHS Substance Abuse and Mental Health Services Administration (SAMHSA). None of our funders, advisers, colleagues, and mentors bears any responsibility for the perspective taken or critiqued here; the authors alone bear that responsibility.

This work is deeply influenced by the understanding gained from, and the mentorship and friendship of two profoundly wonderful women, each of whom created a social movement: Maggie Kuhn, the founder of the Gray Panthers, and Tish Sommers, founder of the Older Women's League.

The most enthusiastic proponent of writing this book was the late Solomon Davis, former graduate student, postdoc, faculty member, and friend. He was coauthor of a previously published earlier version of the chapter on the "Medical-Industrial Complex." That chapter is revised, updated, and expanded here in Chapter 8.

Many colleagues in the Institute of Health and Aging (IHA) at the University of California, San Francisco (UCSF), have contributed in endless ways to making this endeavor possible. Special appreciation is due to Institute Policy Scholar and friend Dixie Horning; to Sheryl

Goldberg, Senior Research Associate, who picked up the pieces and managed and kept the Estes research efforts going through it all; to Martha
Michel, who helped with Social Security and gender data; and to the
countless cohorts of graduate students who took classes taught by
Carroll Estes in Social Policy and Aging, Sociology of Power, Contemporary Social Theory, and Older Women and the State—and who, in
the process, challenged and extended the ideas presented here. Sotiria
Theoharis aided immeasurably with informed theoretical discourses
and her coteaching of the Estes seminar on Contemporary Social
Theory during the final 3 months of "the book." Pre- and postdoctoral
fellows whose work with us over the years contributed are Terry
Arendell, Linda Bergthold, David Carrell, Lita De La Torre, Linda
Facio, Deborah Gerson, Pamela Hanes-Spohn, Robert Hughes, Stan
Ingman, Brian Kaskie, Ellen Morrison, John Oberlander, Stephanie
Robert, Michaela Schunk, Minna Silberberg, Robyn Stone, Andrew
Szasz, Diana Torrez, Toti Villanueva, and Chris Wellin.

The highly competent and continuing assistance of Marie Christine
Yue and Patrick Henderson, Jay Parks, Regina Gudelunas, and Annabel
Paragas, five of the biggest assets of the Institute, kept things on track,
making the book deadlines achievable. Special thanks go to Karen Kerr,
Institute Research Assistant who worked on the earliest draft of what
was to become this book, and Anne Larson, Intern in the UCSF National
Center of Excellence in Women's Health, who relentlessly pursued the
literature and entered and organized references in EndNote. Dawn Ogawa
and Donna Zulman assisted with library searches, special research, and
office management.

Tracy Weitz, analyst and friend, contributed in a myriad of ways,
reading, critiquing, editing, reorganizing, and improving virtually
every part of the book, with particular contributions to Chapters 1, 2,
and 5. Anthony (Tony) Hunter performed miraculously (i.e., calmly,
patiently, and intelligently) in the overall editing of the book at the end
when it seemed too big to finish.

Over the years, Sage Publications has played an important role in
supporting and promoting the publications of Carroll Estes and her
colleagues. This book, the fourth published by Sage, is no exception.
Thanks go to Mitch Allen, who first encouraged our consideration of Sage
in the publication of this and each of the other books that have gone
before: *The Long-Term Care Crisis,* 1993; *Long-Term Care of the Elderly,*

1985; and *Fiscal Austerity and Aging*, 1983. Jim Brace-Thompson, Senior Editor, has "brought the book home" with steady and positive support at every juncture.

Duskie Lynn Estes, Carroll Estes's daughter, was a source of constant support and incentive both to begin and to finish "the book." Carroll's mother, Carroll Cox Estes, an author herself, deserves the credit for teaching Carroll how to write and giving her the courage to do it. Carroll's aunt, Margaret Davis, rendered needed care every step of the process. There is no way such loving contributions can ever be adequately acknowledged.

1 Political Economy of Aging

A Theoretical Framework

Carroll L. Estes

For nearly three decades, application of the political economy perspective has resulted in a more robust understanding of the issues of health and aging by integrating the approaches of economics, political science, sociology, and gerontology, each of which has proven inadequate when employed in isolation. The political economy of aging emphasizes the broad implications of structural forces and processes that contribute to constructions of old age and aging as well as to social policy. It is a systematic view predicated on the assumption that old age can be understood only in the context of social conditions and issues of the larger social order (Estes, 1979; Estes, Gerard, Zones, & Swan, 1984). In addition, the political economy perspective is sensitive to the integral connections between the societal (macrolevel), the organizational and institutional (mesolevel), and the individual (microlevel) dimensions of aging. The framework and approach employed in this volume advance the traditional use of the political economy perspective by refining and expanding prior work done by the author and her colleagues (Estes, 1979, 1999a; Estes, Gerard, Zones, & Swan, 1984). This critical perspective is further informed by new developments in conflict, critical, cultural, and feminist theories (discussed in greater depth in Chapter 2). The theoretical model of the political economy of aging (Figure 1.1) is a multilevel analytical framework that aims to elucidate the socially and structurally produced nature of aging. The conflicting and competitive multidirectional relationships between postindustrial capital, the state, and the sex/gender system

1

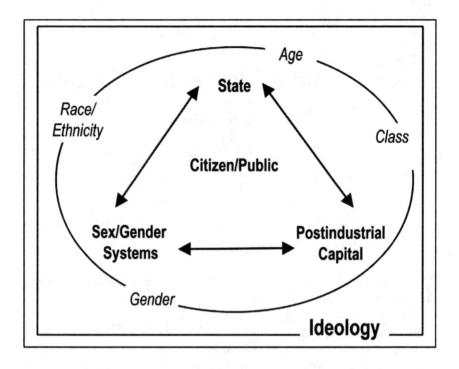

Figure 1.1. Theoretical Political Economy Model: Estes Version

create and incorporate new institutional actors, such as "the medical-industrial complex" and "the aging enterprise." Centered within this model is the public/citizen where the macrolevels and microlevels of analysis are more deeply explored. The power struggles between these institutional forces occur within the context of the "interlocking systems of oppression" (Collins, 1990, 1991) of gender, social class, and racial and ethnic status across the life course (Dressel, Minkler, & Yen, 1999; Street & Quadagno, 1993). Finally, ideology is a key element in defining the issue of aging and determining how policies address aging in society. This chapter explores the unique role that each of these components plays within the theoretical model of social policy and aging. Subsequent chapters explore the complex intersections of these ideas in greater detail.

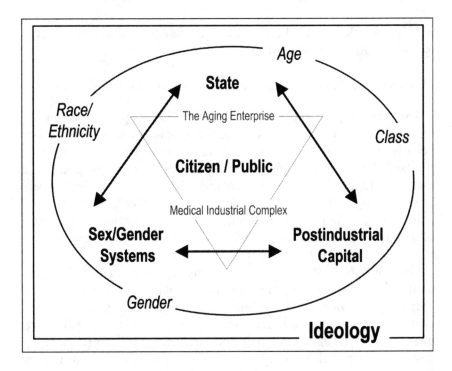

Figure 1.2. Theoretical Model of Social Policy and Aging: Estes Version

Theoretical Model

The Multilevel Analytical Framework

The analytic levels of the framework are (a) financial and post-industrial capital and its globalization, (b) the state, (c) the sex/gender system, and (d) the public and the citizen (see Figure 1.1). For analytic purpose, the model is expanded to include a fifth level—the medical-industrial complex and the aging enterprise (Estes, 1979), which is a product of the relationship between postindustrial capital, the state, and the sex/gender system (see Figure 1.2). Four of the five levels are adapted and revised from McKinlay (1985). According to conflict theory, discussed in detail in Chapter 2, the actors engage in struggles with one another, and policies result from the extent to which one actor is able to dominate and control the others.

Financial and Postindustrial Capital and Its Globalization

The role of capital in the theoretical model for the political economy of aging is well recognized. One of the most salient contemporary debates about financial and postindustrial capital concerns globalization and the relation of old age policy to the economics and politics of markets and the power of corporate capital around the world. Globalization brings with it the processes of privatization, competition, rationalization, and deregulation as well as the transformation of all sectors of society through technology and the flexibilization and deregulation of work (Castells, 1989; Piven & Cloward, 1997).

William Tabb (1999) depicts the perils of monetary globalization, defined as "cross-border movements" of loans, equities, direct and indirect investments, and currencies. He describes a key process of globalization as the "imperialism of finance" in which there are uncontrolled and extraordinarily rapid movements of capital that may destabilize national economies instantly and that may be likened to Keynes's classic discussion of the world ruled by a "parliament of banks." Severe difficulties are inherent in the incapacities of individual nation states to "fix" or "correct" problems that may result from the pressures of financial markets with few controls and little social regulation. When things go wrong, costly bailouts by the state can be expected for financial speculators. Tabb observes that the "logic of [this] financial hegemony" is to "decrease government expenditures and state intervention through privatization and contracting out and do away with capital contributions" (Tabb, 1999, p. 6). This situation produces a "tension between international economic integration and possibilities for progressive politics" (Tabb, 1999, p. 2), the social costs of which are "severe and potentially catastrophic" (Tabb, 1999, p. 3). A case in point in the United States is the pressure to reduce state expenditures and abandon the social contract for the nation's economic and health security to older persons under Social Security and Medicare. The push has been to replace them with privatized programs. This shifts responsibility from the state to the individual, while also reducing corporate contributions, long seen as "deferred wages," to these programs.

The current postindustrial time and space is characterized by the "unfolding of information technology with its unlimited horizons of communication" and control, with "telecommunications reinforcing the commanding role of major business concentrations around the world" and in a social system—capitalism (Castells, 1989, pp. 1-2). Castells (1989) identifies two major macroprocesses that are simultaneously occurring: the "restructuring of capitalism" and "informationalism" (p. 4). He hypothesizes that information technologies influence power exercised both by state institutions and by production and management. Both arenas are crucial in the struggles surrounding the politics of aging, the politics of entitlements, and the politics of race, class, and gender because the United States is in an era of electronically manufactured ("virtual") social movements and the mushrooming of well-funded and conservative think tanks that are applying their media savvy and ingenuity to frame the issues and define the national policy agenda on aging. This combination of capitalism, globalism, and informationalism draws attention to the crucial role of ideological production in U.S. policy debates such as aging. (See the section on ideology in this chapter.)

As a process, debate centers on the "uses" of globalization as the rationale and means by which corporate capital may transnationally pursue new low-wage strategies and weaken the power of labor, women, and minority populations. Globalization extends, perhaps without limits, the corporate capacity of capital to "exit" a nation (and thereby to escape corporate responsibility and/or taxation) in the course of struggles with labor. In this way, globalization offers the possibility of seriously weakening the nation-state. This may be referred to as an opportunity for disciplinary social control of the state by corporate capital—under threat of capital flight elsewhere. At the symbolic and material level, the process of globalization strengthens the irresistibility and power of capital. The inevitability of global market forces and technology challenge the relative power of economics, politics, the state, culture, and social relations more generally.

The State

The state is composed of major social, political, and economic institutions, including the legislative, executive, and judicial branches of government; the military and criminal justice systems; and public educational, health, and welfare institutions (Waitzkin, 1983). See Chapter 4 for an additional discussion of state theory.

Offe and Ronge (1982) identify four characteristics of the state in capitalist societies:

1. Property is private, and privately owned capital is the basis of the economy.
2. Resources generated through private profit and the growth of private wealth indirectly finance the state (e.g., through taxation).
3. The state is thereby "dependent on a source of income which it does not itself organize . . . thus [it] has a general 'interest' in facilitating" the growth of private property in order to perpetuate itself (Giddens & Held, 1982, p. 192).
4. In democracies, political elections disguise the reality that the resources available for distribution by the state are dependent on the success of private profit and capital reinvestment rather than on the will of the electorate.

A fifth attribute of the state is its accountability for the success of the economy; the state bears the brunt of public dissatisfaction for economic difficulties.

O'Connor (1973) and Alford and Friedland (1985) argue that the state in U.S. society has three major functions. First, the state ensures the conditions favorable to economic growth and private profit (allowing for the accumulation of wealth). Second, the state ensures the continuing legitimacy and operation of the social order by alleviating those conditions and problems generated by the free enterprise system (such as unemployment) that might create destructive social unrest. This action is accomplished through the provision of publicly subsidized benefits. Third, the state functions to protect the democratic process (see Chapter 5 for more detail). One problem is that the first two of these functions require the expenditure of public resources. State expenditures that facilitate the accumulation of wealth meet the needs of business and industry through favorable tax treatment and government subsidies: for building industrial parks, for educating and transporting the labor force, and for other investments (such as highways and sewers) that lower production costs. State expenditures for what is traditionally referred to as social welfare reflect the displacement costs of the operation of the economic system—the costs in poverty, sexism, racism, and ageism.

The tension created by the demand for these two different types of expenditures (favorable treatment for business and social welfare) often results in a propensity for the state to spend itself into fiscal crisis. Eventually, this forces the state's necessary retreat from the fiscal underwriting of the costs of one or both of these functions (O'Connor, 1973). Furthermore, as capitalist industry gets larger and more monopolistic in character, moves into international markets, and advances technologically, the costs of capital formation and reinvestment increase. At the same time, there are increased demands on the state for assistance in meeting those costs (tax subsidies, roads, bridges, toxic waste cleanups, etc.). Although the state subsidizes more of the costs, the benefits of the investments continue to be returned as private profit. In conjunction, because monopoly is not labor intensive, workers are pushed into a diminishing competitive sector. This exacerbates unemployment and increases the need for state subsidies to alleviate the cumulative negative consequences of these processes. From a political economy perspective, the dual functions of public spending are of the utmost importance because the size of the federal budget is viewed not only in nominal terms but also in terms of the complex and competitive interaction between the public and the private sectors of the economy.

Theorists explicitly working on old age and the state include a list of distinguished scholars.[1] In a theoretical model for social policy and aging, analysis at the level of the state investigates questions regarding the state's role in social provision for the aged, in light of the state's power to (a) allocate and distribute scarce resources, (b) mediate between different segments and classes of society, and (c) alleviate conditions that potentially threaten the social order. Quadagno (1999a) describes the recent shift in the United States to a "capital investment state" characterized by the restructuring of public benefits to coincide with interests of the private sector; the transfer of responsibility from government to the individual and family; and the shift from cash benefits to incentives for saving.

Analysis of public policy directing the allocation and distribution of resources for the nation's older citizens needs to go beyond the scarcity model. It is not merely a question of whether there are enough resources to support domestic social spending. The more important issue is the actual and perceived impact that allocating an increasing share of resources to the aged has on business and economic growth and on the relations of industry and labor (Myles, 1984). The essential issue, from a political economy perspective, concerns the effect that public spending has on the functions of the private economy in terms of ensuring and maintaining a flow of capital for profits and investments. Conservative economists, for example, have charged that Social Security has reduced the public's reliance on the market, increased the individual's dependency on government, and reduced incentives for personal savings, which are a major source of the investment capital essential for economic growth (Rahn & Simonson, 1980). The economic significance of the "graying of America" is that

> it increases the size of the public economy and reduces the share of the national income directly subject to market forces. Thus, while population aging is unlikely to break the "national bank" it will alter the bank's structure of ownership and control. (Myles, 1982, p. 19)

Ultimately, how many resources are controlled by the state or the private economy is a political decision. The relative amounts allocated to supporting the supply of capital (for reinvestment and profit) and to workers or to social welfare costs are never set. However, these allocations are constantly subject to political and economic struggle. Domestic social spending for the needs of income and health compete with other political priorities.

The Sex/Gender System

The third level of the analytic framework advanced in this chapter, the sex/gender system, is a recent addition to the political economy discussion. Although prior work has examined the role of gender at the individual and policy levels, the inclusion of the sex/gender system in the framework as one of the key institutional forces in explaining social policy on aging is new. Prior work of feminist scholars used the term patriarchy to describe the institution of male domination that accompanies the symbolic male principle (Kramarae & Treichler, 1992; Rowbotham, 1981). However, patriarchy has been used to refer more specifically to those relationships at the level of the family, whereas the phrase "sex/gender system" has been proposed to refer to the larger context of male domination and the structures that create and promote domination.[2]

According to Gayle Rubin (1975), the sex/gender system is a set of arrangements by which society transforms biological sexuality into products of human activity and in which these transformed sexual needs are satisfied. The sex/gender system is reflected in social institutions such as the state and the family (Acker, 1988) and in how these "gendered institutions" (Acker, 1992) reproduce the subordination of women (Hartmann, 1981; Walby, 1986) and reinforce women's subjugation (Acker, 1992) through institutions such as marriage and kinship (Rubin, 1975). Old age policy is one of those institutions.

Joan Acker (1988) observes that understanding "class and gender discrimination and exploitation [is] integral to understanding the oppression of women in industrial capitalist societies" (p. 473). She also argues that the relations that produce class are gendered processes, structured through relations of distribution as well as relations of production. Personal relations (particularly marriage), wages, and the state are each locations of gendered distribution that are vitally affected by the dominance of market relations as the basis of distribution. The material base of patriarchy thus rests on the social relations between men and women (Walby, 1986) and the significant material consequences in the form of inequality by gender in old age that flows from those relations. These social relations are expressed in the family and marriage, in the workforce, in the state, and in the roles and social relations that women have within these institutions.

It is widely argued by feminist scholars that the state is a major vehicle for the subjugation of women (Acker, 1988; Connell, 1987; MacKinnon, 1989; Sassoon, 1987b) and that the state is in itself a patriarchal institution. (See Chapter 6 for a discussion of the gendered nature of state policy for the elderly and an examination of the resulting gender inequalities.) Wendy Brown (1995) argues that female subjects are produced by the state through (a) the regulation of pornography and reproduction and (b) women's dependence on the state for survival. Brown and others make the point that because of the gendered state, women's dependency has shifted from the men to the state (Brown, 1995) and from the family to the state (Dickinson & Russell, 1986; Estes, 1991a, 1998a, 1998b; Orloff, 1993). According to Brown (1995), women face the "rational unfreedom regulated by the state" versus their state of "nature" in which there is arbitrary violence by men against them as women. The state meets the requirement of men to protect women from the violence that men cause. The role of dependency in the health and aging of women is explored in greater detail in both Chapter 6 and Chapter 7.

The Citizen and the Public

At the level of the citizen and the public, the framework incorporates an examination of the meaning of citizenship and the rights and benefits of citizens granted by the state through public policy. Both have significant effects on older individuals and the public. These effects vary substantially depending on social class, gender, and racial and ethnic status. The approach builds on a critical literature on citizenship that challenges the uniform (i.e., white male) experience of citizenship as universally and equally shared (O'Connor, Orloff, & Shaver, 1999; Sassoon, 1991; Taylor, 1996; Twine, 1994). Sassoon's proscription is to "historicize and make concrete the concept of citizenship," which is a highly complex and differentiated relationship to the state, mediated through a wide range of institutions. In these institutions, the differences between people, according to resources and needs, family situation and point in the life cycle, and life history with regard to the world of work are as significant as equality before the law or equal political rights (Sassoon, 1991, p. 90). The approach is consistent with feminist and antiracist critiques that

> go beyond a claim for equal opportunities [and are]. . . informed by the recognition of the differentiated effects of an equal application of the rules to people who are different. On the one hand, this is because the rules themselves contain assumptions that are far from neutral or universal. On the other hand, the very notion of the universal in silencing differences in fact derives its very meaning from subordinating or marginalizing the other, the specific, the particular, the different. (Sassoon, 1991, p. 98)

A serious problem is that in capitalist democracies the tension between capitalism and democracy produces a basic dilemma and contradiction surrounding citizenship (Alford & Friedland, 1985; Myles, 1984). Formally, "citizenship is indifferent to economic standing. . . . Yet in capitalist societies where the state protects property, citizenship and class are not easily separable" (Plotkin & Scheuerman, 1994, p. 29). The difficulty is that

> political democracy, meaning governance by the economic majority, represents a real threat to the rich. A strong pro-democratic government, one that governs in the interest of the economic majority, is empowered to tax and regulate business; to redistribute and reallocate power and wealth; to use deficit spending as a tool of economic management and social justice; to bring pressure on business elites to use their wealth in the interest of the vast majority.... The closest that working people can come to power of the economy is in their powers to tax and set the priorities of public spending. If it means anything, after all, democracy means the power of the people themselves to direct how taxes will be raised and spent, without being led around by elites who regularly urge people to think and care about what elites think they ought to care about. (Plotkin & Scheuerman, 1994, p. 29)

How public policy defines citizen rights is highly determinative of the "life chances" available to members of society, including the elderly. In liberal states such as the United States, there are modest universal transfers and means-tested assistance with strict entitlement rules, often associated with stigma (Esping-Andersen, 1990). In contrast to the "largely individualistic and sometimes asocial views of the New Right" in which citizen rights are based largely on labor market participation and property, the opposing concept of "social rights" emphasizing notions of interdependence and solidarity (Twine, 1994) is consistent with the critical perspective proposed here.

The concept of social rights of citizenship is "grounded in the notion of 'lifecourse interdependence' " (Twine, 1994, p. 28). Indeed, "quality of life in old age strongly reflects the different costs of 'lifecourse interdependencies,' of child rearing and employment, and these vary by social class and gender" (Twine, 1994, p. 34). The neoliberal ideology of individualism supports the concept that we are independent, as if independent of society, "a form of freedom from society or more specifically freedom from the state" (Twine, 1994, p. 9). The reluctance to accept our "interdependence" stems from the fact that doing so "would present us with moral obligations to compensate those who bear the costs of our progress" (Twine, 1994, p. 29). A critical approach to social policy and aging assumes that "the material and human reproduction of society involves relations and processes of interdependence" (Twine, 1994, p. 29). Hence, it is appropriate for social policy on aging to reflect these life course and society-wide interdependencies.

The Medical-Industrial Complex and the Aging Enterprise

The social relations between the state, postindustrial capital, the sex/gender system, and the public/citizen have fueled the creation and growth of the medical-industrial complex (Ehrenreich & Ehrenreich, 1971; Estes, Harrington, & Pellow, 2000; Relman, 1980) and the aging enterprise in the United States (Estes, 1979). Central to both the medical-industrial complex and the aging enterprise is the commodification of health that transformed health care and the needs of the elderly and others in society into commodities for specific economic markets (Estes, 1979). What is most relevant to the concern for health and aging is that "business and government . . . look at medical care as more nearly an economic product than a social good" (Iglehart, 1982, p. 120). Within this context, the incentive is to maximize profits rather than health. The consequences for the elderly (as well as for all persons dependent on public policy and programs) are that social needs are turning into profit-making commodities (Scull, 1977). The needs of the elderly are defined and processed by the medical-industrial complex in ways that serve to medicalize old age further and to exacerbate rather than alleviate the dependency of the elderly (Estes & Binney, 1989). The creation of the aging enterprise reflects an aspect of this trend (Estes, 1979, 1986a).

A consideration is how state policies define and commodify the problems of aging. Policies define the problems as individual medical problems requiring medical services sold privately for profit. This approach is ideologically and practically consistent with the state's dual and contradictory roles in promoting the process of capital accumulation and in the legitimation of capitalist social relations through safety net and other provisions (Estes, 1979; Estes, Gerard, Zones, & Swan, 1984; O'Connor, 1973). Because U.S. state policy supports the accumulation function through the gigantic and highly profitable medical-industrial complex (Estes, Harrington, & Pellow, 2000), the "problems of old age" are defined largely at the individual rather than the social or structural level. Furthermore, the "problem" is constructed in ways that emphasize the need for a medical service industry and individual behavior changes to promote successful aging rather than a right to a living wage or adequate income or housing.

Inclusion of the medical-industrial complex and the aging enterprise in the proposed theoretical model of social policy and aging draws attention to health and long-term care policy as products of the relations between the state, capital, and the sex and gender system. Highlighted are key trends in market-driven reform and restructuring, the growth of proprietary care, corporate mergers, and for-profit managed care corporations. On the long-term care side, trends include the commodification of aging (Estes, 1979), privatization, competition, rationalization, devolution, informalization, medicalization (Estes & Binney, 1989), and institutionalization (Estes, Swan, & associates, 1993). Each of these trends has vitally shaped the resources available to and the life chances of elders under old age policy. An in-depth discussion of this level of the framework is provided in Chapter 8.

The Interlocking Systems of Oppression

Over the past decade, there has been increased acknowledgment of the multiplier and layering effects of race/ethnicity, gender, class, and age, postulated as the interlocking systems of oppression (Collins, 1990, 1991). Collins makes a conceptual distinction between interlocking oppression and intersectionality, arguing that gender, race, and class across the life span are different but interrelated axes of social structure not just features of experience.

First, the notion of interlocking oppression refers to the macrolevel connections linking systems of oppression such as race, class, and gender. This is the model describing the social structure that creates social positions. Second, the notion of intersectionality describes microlevel processes—namely, how each individual and group occupies a social position with interlocking structures of oppression described by the metaphor or intersectionality. Together they shape oppression (Collins, 1991)

The political economy model illuminates how social policy for the aged mirrors the structural arrangements of U.S. society and the distribution of material, political, and symbolic resources within it. Social class, race/ethnicity, and gender are seen as directly related to the resources on which persons may draw in old age (Estes, Gerard, Zones, & Swan, 1984).

Social Class

The role of social class is well established in the political economy model. Public policy reflects and reinforces the "life chances" associated with each person's social location within the class, status, and political structures that make up society (Weber, 1946). What is emphasized here is greater comprehension of the relationship between social class and the unique, but interconnected, phenomena experienced and social systems encompassed in the concepts of race/ethnicity, gender, and generation. Class analysis is concerned with relative control over policy, resources, and other people. Broadly speaking, class analysis calls attention to class structure, class formation, class struggle, and class consciousness, examining the interconnections between these levels and their implications for social policy in old age (Wright, 1997). Preretirement class is a major factor affecting postretirement conditions of the elderly. Estes has argued that

> current old age policy in the United States reflects a two-tiered system of welfare with benefits distributed on the basis of legitimacy rather than need (Tussing, 1971). Old age neither levels nor diminishes social class distinctions (Crystal, 1982; Estes, 1982; Nelson, 1982). It is the individual lifetime conditions and labor force participation established before retirement age that largely determine an older person's social class and economic resources....We recognize class . . . is much more complex than income status alone. (Estes, Gerard, Zones, & Swan, 1984, p. 100)

The structural dependency of the aged as a group and as individuals "arises from conditions in the labor market and in the stratification of work and society" (Estes, Gerard, Zones, & Swan, 1984, p. 31). The concept of "deservingness" incorporated into the design of old age policies is firmly rooted in the principle of differential rewards for differential achievements during a lifetime (Nelson, 1982; Townsend, 1981; Tussing, 1971). Those seen as "deserving" are recipients of mainstream social insurance programs such as Social Security, and those who are seen as "undeserving" are the poor and low-income persons who are outside of or marginal to the mainstream labor force participation. These people become recipients of social assistance largely through stigmatizing means-tested programs such as Supplemental Security Income and Medicaid that vary from state to state.

Krieger and colleagues argue that the increasing social inequalities in health in the United States, coupled with growing inequalities in income and wealth, have refocused attention on social class as a key determinant of population health (Krieger, Williams, & Moss, 1997). A growing body of evidence indicates that socioeconomic status (SES) is a strong predictor of health, regardless of access to medical care. SES continues to be a remarkably robust indicator of rates of illness and death (Williams & Collins, 1995), and numerous studies and reviews have demonstrated this conclusion (Adler et al., 1994; Adler, Boyce, Chesney, Folkman, & Syme, 1993; Adler & Coriell, 1997; Krieger, Rowley, Herman, Avery, & Phillips, 1993; Lantz et al., 1998). The relationship between SES and health occurs at every socioeconomic level and for a broad range of SES indicators and cannot be accounted for simply by classic risk factors such as diet and smoking (Adler et al., 1993). The relationship is so strong that each level of SES is associated with better health outcomes. This occurrence, although not completely understood, is referred to as the "SES gradient in health status" (Adler et al., 1994; Adler et al., 1993).

Race/Ethnicity

Although race and ethnicity are deeply interconnected to social class, it is essential to understand that they are distinctly separate from social class. Williams (1996) offers a strong and persuasive critique of the limited and inadequate treatment of race and racism by theorists of the welfare state, including scholars using the critical approaches of political economy and feminism. The analytical framework described in this chapter incorporates an analysis of race and racism as part of understanding the origins and consequences of old age policy (see Quadagno, 1994). Welfare state policy is inextricably linked with race through global processes such as imperialism and immigration policies that have facilitated the exploitation and oppression of blacks and other minorities (Williams, 1996).

Current research has shown race/ethnicity to be independent of socioeconomic status as a risk factor for poorer health outcomes (Gornick et al., 1996). Race and racism affect populations in differing ways depending on the experience and relationship with the dominant culture. As such, it is critical to acknowledge both the existence of institutional racism within social structures and power relations and its independent and interlocking effects on old age and aging policy. A more complete discussion of the role of race/ethnicity in health and aging is provided in Chapter 7.

Scholars have argued for a wider conceptualization of the processes through which racism is linked to ill health and thus an understanding of the effects of racism at the political, socioeconomic, community, and family levels (McKenzie, 1998). Through a review of the literature, McKenzie (1998) argues that racism produces its effects through segregation, socioeconomic stratification, and marginalization as well as through the individual experience. Krieger (1999) has written extensively on the impact of racism and discrimination on health, arguing that both the economic consequences of discrimination and accumulated insults arising from everyday experience and violence are major health issues. Employing an ecosocial framework, she and her colleagues have documented patterns of discrimination within the United States. Institutionalized racism produces discriminatory effects on health through public policy, the physical environment, social and medical services, and preventive health policy (McKenzie, 1998). King has developed a conceptual framework for understanding and applying the concept of institutional racism to the health care system (King, 1996).

Gender

A major underdeveloped area of great significance in the political economy of aging concerns the differential gendered consequences of aging from a life course perspective. Historically, theories of the state and class fail to explicitly and adequately address the subordination of women and the privileging of men (Acker, 1988). Acker (1992) contends that gender is a dimension of domination and discrimination that is neither obviously discrete nor structurally analogous to social class or race/ethnicity. She argues that because the state, the economy, and other institutions have been developed and dominated by men and thus symbolically interpreted from the standpoint of men, these institutions are defined by the absence of women (Acker, 1992). The incorporation of gender into the theoretical model offers the opportunity to better understand how the status of women is created and reinforced by political and economic structures and how the effects of social class and race/ethnicity are exacerbated for women. Finally, it is important to understand that gender plays a separate yet defining role in the influence of age.

Women constitute an increasing segment of the aging population. O'Rand (1996) argues that the older population of the United States is undergoing a feminization. Despite their increased longevity, older women live under more compromised circumstances than those experienced by men. In general, older women are more likely than men to live in poverty, to have less access to a secure retirement, and to pay an increased percentage of their income on out-of-pocket health care costs. Likewise, women play substantially different social roles than men, and those roles directly affect their health and economic well-being. Women are also more likely than men to suffer from chronic conditions and disabilities that limit their quality of life (Rice & Michel, 1998). Prior work of Estes and Weitz (2000) has hypothesized that these outcomes result from the role of gender in social and political structures and processes. Four aspects of this influence are notable:

1. There is a gendered relationship between socioeconomic structures and health over time.
2. There are gender-specific implications of health care financing and policy.
3. There is a gender bias in the disease-based medical model of health.
4. There are health consequences to the gendered nature of caregiving.

Ideology

As belief systems, ideologies are competing worldviews that reflect the social position and structural advantages of their adherents. All political and economic regimes use ideology as the discourse with which to communicate and impose a reflection of the dominant social relations. The perspective advanced here concurs with Therborn's (1980) in rejecting the narrow definition of ideology as false beliefs that may be contrasted with scientific truth or intellectual doctrinal systems. As described by Thompson (1986), Therborn's view is that "Ideologies are social phenomena of a discursive type, including both everyday notions and experience, and elaborate intellectual doctrines; both the consciousness of social actors and the institutionalized thought systems and discourses of a given society" (Thompson, 1986, p. 15).

Ideology is integral to the three processes by which dominant views of social policy and aging are produced and sustained:

1. The successful creation of cultural images by policymakers, experts, and the media—for example, that the elderly are "greedy geezers"
2. The appeal to the necessities of the economic system—for example, claiming that the elderly are responsible for the nation's economic problems by "busting the budget"
3. The implementation of policy and the application of expertise in ways that transform conflicts over goals and means into systems of rational problem solving

This focus on rational problem resolution by technical experts serves to obfuscate the substance of class, gender, and racial/ethnicity (George & Wilding as cited in Manning, 1985) inherent in both the definition of the problem and the "solutions" that attend to those definitions. An example is the purportedly "gender neutral" policy of Social Security that presently is biased toward the autonomous nuclear family. Ideologies of the state, the market, and the sex/gender system have tremendous consequences, particularly for those that are most dependent on the state—women, minorities, the poor, the elderly, and the disabled.

In considering social policy on aging, the challenges with regard to ideology are (a) to locate the systems of beliefs and values within specific social formations (such as old age policy) and examine how they articulate with the economic system of capitalism, the state, and class and other gender and race struggles therein and (b) to investigate these ideological communities, which exist within specific organized collectivities (e.g., nation-states, organizations, institutions) and how they mask past social and class struggles and contradictory norms and values (Thompson, 1986, p. 14).

Conclusion

The work from critical perspectives on aging, particularly that on the political economy of aging, has attracted the attention of an increasing number of scholars. Fueled by a growing awareness of the global economy that is shaping every aspect of U.S. economy and society as well as the fate of all age cohorts, scholars are paying increased attention to the conflict between the state and postindustrial capital. Layoffs, work outsourcing to other nations, the growing concentration of capital with corporate mergers and restructuring, the diminishing number and influence of union members, and declining wages and employee benefits have raised profound fears among millions of working Americans about their job security and their standards of living. The gap between rich and poor grows wider, and millions in the middle class now experience working class uncertainty. These class struggles are exacerbated by struggles around gender, race/ethnicity, and age, all of which are reinforced through ideology and fuel the construction of social policy on aging.

The theoretical model for social policy and aging presented in this chapter provides a framework to understand and analyze these struggles. Based on the political economy perspective, the model uses a multilevel analytical framework that addresses the conflicting and competitive multidirectional and recursive relationships between postindustrial capital, the state, and the sex/gender system, which create and support the medical-industrial complex and the aging enterprise. The role of the public/citizen is also explored, and macrolevels, mesolevels, and microlevels of analysis are included. The model recognizes that the power struggles between actors occur within the context of the "interlocking systems of oppression" of gender, social class, and racial and ethnic status across the life course. Last, power struggles over ideology reflect the dominant social relations and provide the environmental context for defining the issues of old age and aging and determining how policies address these phenomena in society.

Notes

1. The following are examples of theorists' work on old age and the state.

Theorists from the United Kingdom:

Phillipson, C. (1982). *Capitalism and the construction of old age*. London: Macmillan.
Phillipson, C. (1998). *Reconstructing old age: New agendas in social theory and practice*. London: Sage.
Townsend, P. (1981). The structured dependency of the elderly: A creation of social policy in the twentieth century. *Ageing and Society*, 1(1), 5-28.

Walker, A. (1980). Social creation of poverty and dependency in old age. *Journal of Social Policy, 9*(1), 49-75.

Walker, A. (1981). Towards a political economy of old age. *Ageing and Society, 1*(1), 73-94.

Walker, A. (1991). *Intergenerational relations and welfare restructuring: The social construction of a generational problem.* Paper presented at the Conference on the New Contract Between the Generations: Social Science Perspectives on Cohorts in the 21st Century, University of Southern California, Los Angeles, CA.

Walker, A. (1999). Public policy and theories of aging: Constructing and reconstructing old age. In V. Bengston & K. Schaie (Eds.), *Handbook of theories of aging* (pp. 361-378). New York: Springer.

John Myles in Canada and the United States:

Myles, J. (1984). *Old age in the welfare state: The political economy of public pensions.* Boston: Little Brown.

Myles, J. (1991). Postwar capitalism and the extension of Social Security into a retirement wage. In M. Minkler & C. L. Estes (Eds.), *Critical perspectives on aging: The political and moral economy of growing old* (pp. 293-309). Amityville, NY: Baywood.

Myles, J., & Quadagno, J. S. (1991). *States, labor markets, and the future of old age policy.* Philadelphia: Temple University Press.

Myles, J. F. (1996). When markets fail: Social welfare in Canada and the United States. In G. Esping-Andersen (Ed.), *Welfare states in transition: National adaptations in global economies* (pp. 116-140). London: Sage.

The work of Estes and colleagues in the United States:

Estes, C. L. (1979). *The aging enterprise.* San Francisco: Jossey-Bass.

Estes, C. L. (1980). Constructions of reality. *Journal of Social Issues, 36*(2), 117-132.

Estes, C. L. (1986a). The aging enterprise: In whose interests. *International Journal of Health Services, 16*(2), 243-251.

Estes, C. L. (1986b). The politics of ageing in America. *Ageing and Society, 6,* 121-134.

Estes, C. L. (1991a). The new political economy of aging: Introduction and critique. In M. Minkler & C. L. Estes (Eds.), *Critical perspectives on aging: The political and moral economy of growing old* (pp. 19-36). Amityville, NY: Baywood.

Estes, C. L. (1991b). The Reagan legacy: Privatization, the welfare state, and aging in the 1990s. In J. Myles & J. S. Quadagno (Eds.), *States, labor markets, and the future of old age policy* (pp. 59-83). Philadelphia: Temple University Press.

Estes, C. L. (1999). Critical gerontology and the new political economy of aging. In M. Minkler & C. L. Estes (Eds.), *Critical gerontology: Perspectives from political and moral economy* (pp. 17-35). Amityville, NY: Baywood.

Estes, C. L., Gerard, L., & Clarke, A. (1984). Women and the economics of aging. *International Journal of Health Services, 14*(1), 55-68.

Estes, C. L., Gerard, L., Zones, J. S., & Swan, J. (1984). *Political economy, health, and aging.* Boston: Little Brown.

Estes, C. L., Linkins, K. W., & Binney, E. A. (1996). The political economy of aging. In R. H. Binstock & L. K. George (Eds.), *Handbook of aging and the social sciences* (pp. 346-361). San Diego, CA: Academic Press.

Estes, C. L., Swan, J. H., & Gerard, L. (1982). Dominant and competing paradigms: Toward a political economy of aging. *Ageing and Society, 2*(2), 151-164.

Jill Quadagno and colleagues in the United States:

Quadagno, J. S. (1989). Generational equity and the politics of the welfare state. *Politics & Society, 17*(3), 353-377.

Quadagno, J. S. (1988). *The transformation of old age security: Class and politics in the American welfare state.* Chicago: University of Chicago Press.

Street, D., & Quadagno, J. S. (1993). The state, the elderly, and the intergenerational contract: Toward a new political economy of aging. In K. Schaie & A. Achenbaum (Eds.), *Societal impact on aging* (pp. 130-150). New York: Springer.

Others in the United States:

Calasanti, T., & Zajicek, A. (1993). A socialist feminist approach to aging: Embracing diversity. *Journal of Aging Studies, 7*(2), 117-131.

Harrington Meyer, M. (1990). Family status and poverty among older women: The gendered distribution of retirement income in the U.S. *Social Problems, 37*(4), 551-563.

Harrington Meyer, M. (1996). Making claims as workers or wives: The distribution of Social Security benefits. *American Sociological Review, 61*(3), 449-465.

Olson, L. K. (1994). Women and social security: A progressive approach. *Journal of Aging and Social Policy, 6,* 43-56.

Pampel, F. C. (1994). Population aging, class context, and age inequality in public spending. *American Journal of Sociology, 100*(1), 153-196.

Pampel, F. C., & Williamson, J. B. (1989). *Age, class, politics, and the welfare state.* New York: Cambridge University Press.

Pampel, F. C., & Williamson, J. (1995). Age structure, politics and cross national patterns of public pension expenditures. *American Sociological Review, 50,* 787-798.

Skocpol, T. (1992). *Protecting soldiers and mothers: The political origins of social policy in the United States.* Cambridge, MA: Belknap Press of Harvard University Press.

In France:

Guillemard, A. M. (1993). Older workers and the labour market. In A. Walker, J. Alber, & A. M. Guillemard (Eds.), *Older people in Europe: Social and economic policies* (pp. 35-51). Brussels: Commission on the European Communities.

Kohli, M., Guillemard, A. M., & Gunsteren, H. V. (Eds.). (1991). *Time for retirement: Comparative studies of early exit from the labour force.* Cambridge, MA: Cambridge University Press.

2. This volume has adopted the phrase "sex/gender system" for the theoretical model, while acknowledging that many feminist scholars still use the term *patriarchy* to refer to the larger system of male oppression. Integrity of terms with other authors' original works is therefore maintained in the interchangeability of terms within this discussion.

2 Critical Perspectives on Aging

Carroll L. Estes
Karen W. Linkins
Elizabeth A. Binney

As interest in social policy and the aging of the population has intensified in Europe and the United States in the past decade, old age
and aging have been constructed and regarded as a problem of the
welfare state. The policy focus of Western industrialized nations has
centered on the role of the welfare state in the financing of care and
support for the elderly (Kohli, 1988). A critical perspective on social
policy and aging challenges dominant and mainstream thinking in
gerontology that tends to reduce aging to an individual problem of
dependency while overlooking broad social, economic, and political
factors and structural arrangements integral to (and that in some ways
actually "produce") old age and aging as it is known (Estes, 1979). With
reductionist and individualistic approaches, significant aspects of
aging are underexplored, such as the meaning and lived experience of
old age and the aging process as well as the dynamics of inequality
within the aging population. These dynamics include differences in old
age by race, class, and gender. Another particularly underdeveloped
dimension of social policy is work on how the state and the economy

AUTHORS' NOTE: Some material in this chapter is adapted from "Critical Perspectives on Health
and Aging," by C. L. Estes and K. W. Linkins. In *Handbook of Social Studies in Health and Medicine*,
edited by G. L. Albrecht, R. Fitzpatrick, and S. C. Scrimshaw (pp. 154-172). (London: Sage, 2000).

(capital) are organized and function to produce the individual and aggregate outcomes.

This chapter begins with a discussion of prevailing gerontological theories and their limitations as contrasted with the critical approach proposed here. The subsequent section introduces the theoretical roots of the critical perspective and the sources of the increased interest in this work during the past four decades. A discussion follows of the four major theoretical perspectives that make up work from critical perspectives: (a) conflict theories, (b) critical theories, (c) feminist theories, and (d) cultural studies. Finally, the critical theoretical approach is applied to gerontology under the topics of the political economy of aging and cultural studies in aging, such as moral economy and humanistic gerontology. A discussion of the role of ideology accompanies this application.

Prevailing Gerontological Theories and Their Limitations

Since its inception in 1945, the field of gerontology has evolved into a formal interdisciplinary science involving biology, clinical medicine, and the behavioral and social sciences. Although researchers, practitioners, and the general public agree that aging is a part of the life course, there has been substantial disagreement among and within these groups regarding the definition of old age, the perception of what constitutes normal aging, and the extent and scope of public/private responsibility for optimal, successful, or productive aging. This disparity in perspectives is reflected in the broad and fragmented body of theory that constitutes the field of gerontology where "there is no common thread or tie to a common core of disciplinary knowledge to unify the field" (Estes, Binney, & Culbertson, 1992, p. 50).

One dimension of this fragmented body of work on aging stems from the larger social science debate between "micro" versus "macro" perspectives in which the leading theories of aging emphasize either the individual actor or the structure of society as the primary object of study. A small number of theoretical strands attempt to link both microperspectives and macroperspectives (Bengtson, Burgess, & Parrott, 1997; Marshall, 1996). Newer efforts have attempted also to integrate the mesoperspective (Estes, 1998b). Another classification dimension of different gerontological theories (also consistent with the larger disciplinary social sciences) is the "normative" versus the "interpretive" perspective (Hendricks, 1992; Marshall, 1996). A third classification dimension that may be contrasted with the previous two is the "critical," or "radical," perspective.

Many of the leading theories of aging, especially those that approach the study of aging from the perspectives of biology and social psychology, focus on the *individual as the primary unit of analysis.* In the early work (1945 to the 1980s), the aging process was most often viewed and assessed in terms of the biological breakdown of the individual, or in terms of the individual personality and process, and the presumed concomitant dependency, loss, and requisite adjustment to these states of being.

Disengagement Theory

The "first generation" of gerontological theories (Bengtson et al., 1997; Hendricks, 1992) developed by social psychologists focused on the individual, culminating in disengagement theory and activity theory. Disengagement theory (Cumming & Henry, 1961) posits that old age is a period in which the aging individual and society both simultaneously engage in mutual separation (e.g., retirement and disengagement from the workforce). The process of disengagement is treated as a natural, universal, biologically based, and normal part of the life course. This assertion also fits into the broader functionalist paradigm that was dominant at the time of its development (late 1950s–late 1960s) in which disengagement was presumed to be "functional" from the standpoints of both the individual and society. Although disengagement theory is no longer widely accepted among researchers in aging, its influence is still apparent in the policy arena. Social Security and Medicare as well as the retirement policies in the private sector are all policies based in an acceptance of disengagement theory. In fact, disengagement theory provides a theoretical rationale for the trend in implementing incentives for early retirement in private and public sector institutions that have been promoted over the past several decades.

Activity Theory

Activity theory developed in opposition to the assumptions of disengagement theory, asserting that people in old age continue the roles and activities they have developed over the course of life, including maintaining the same needs and values present at earlier points in their lives. The basic assumption of this theory is that the more active people are, the more likely they are to be satisfied with their lives. Activity theory stimulated the development of several social psychological theories of aging, including continuity theory (Costa & McCrae, 1980) and successful aging (Abeles, Gift, & Ory, 1994; Baltes & Baltes, 1990; Rowe & Kahn, 1987). Drawn from developmental or life cycle theory (Lowenthal, 1975; Neugarten, 1964), continuity theory asserts that aging persons have the need and the tendency to maintain the same personalities, habits, and perspectives that they developed over the life course. An individual who is successfully aging maintains a mature integrated personality, which also is the basis of life satisfaction (Neugarten, Havinghurst, & Tobin, 1968). As such, decreases in activity or social interaction are viewed as related more to changes in health and physical function than to an inherent need for a shift in or relinquishment of previous roles. The continuing focus on individual aging brings with it certain problems.

Successful and Productive Aging

More recently developed theories of successful aging expand the basic framework of activity and continuity theory to three fundamental components: low probability of disease and disease-related disability, high cognitive and physical functional capacity, and active engagement with life (Rowe & Kahn, 1997). In the 1990s, successful-aging theories reemerged but were seen as involving more than the absence of disease and more than the maintenance of functional capacities. Instead, these two components combine and interact with the active engagement of life. A related theoretical development is the area of "productive aging," which is similar to the work on successful aging, and seeks to promote a positive image of aging through the redefinition of and continuing "productivity" of older individuals. Critics (Holstein, 1992; see also Estes, Mahakian, & Weitz, Chapter 9, this volume) note that the productive aging framework places responsibility on the individual (and individual health behaviors) and may also create expectations for "work" (especially for women) for many years, often without pay and through the end of life. In conjunction, the health and economic liabilities associated with race, class, and gender that would justify policies and programs to compensate for these inequalities, and the physical and mental stresses associated with them, are ignored.

On the surface, activity theory and its later derivations of successful and productive aging promote the eradication of ageist stereotypes of the elderly and create opportunities for individual empowerment and quality of life in later years. Nevertheless, these theories take little account of the influence of structural factors on individual outcomes, nor do they suggest what to do about race, gender, and class as crucial social mediators of the experience of aging successfully and productively. In addition, such theories provide little insight for understanding the broader (and unequal) division of labor (including women's significant unpaid caregiving burden across the life course) and the growing disparities in the allocation of resources across groups in society. Thus, policies and programs developed from these theories are not likely to address the pervasive structural basis of diversity and heterogeneity of the aging experience. They do not address social inequalities in health or any other aspect of old age.

Increasingly, gerontological scholars acknowledge the malleability and reversibility of various biological and behavioral phenomena that were previously thought to be inevitable with age (Rowe & Kahn, 1987, 1998). There is also a growing recognition of the influence of social, behavioral, and environmental factors in explaining the processes of aging and of health in old age (House, Kessler, & Herzog, 1990). The formidable environmental barriers to health and healthy behaviors and lifestyles (e.g., safety and economic security and even racial segregation) in poor urban inner-city neighborhoods have been shown to produce independent negative health outcomes (Collins & Williams, 1999; Robert, 1999).

This work is consistent with a long-standing and substantial body of literature affirming the import of social, behavioral, and environmental factors in both individual and population health more generally (Adler, Boyce, Chesney, Folkman, & Syme, 1993; Geiger, 1981; Hahn & Kaplan, 1985; McGinnis & Foege, 1993; McKeown, 1978; Navarro, 1990; Syme & Berkman, 1976). Epidemiologist John Cassell and his colleagues (Geiger, 1981) have identified three important principles governing the relationships between *changes* in the social, biological, and physical environments and the likelihood of increased incidence of disease (e.g., strokes, hypertension, tuberculosis, and coronary heart disease): (a) social and family disorganization (with more disorganization leading to more negative health outcomes), (b) domination and subordination (with the more dominant showing the least deleterious health effects and those who are subordinate having the most extreme responses), and (c) the presence and effectiveness of buffers or protective factors such as group or social supports (with those who are more supported being more protected).

Specifically related to aging, Bortz and Bortz (1996) and Rowe and Kahn (1987, 1998) suggest the declining significance of medical and biological factors in health with advancing age. Riley and Riley (1994a) highlight the interplay of social structures (structural opportunities in schools, offices, families, communities, social networks, and society at large) and structural change in the explanation of healthy and successful aging. Others have calculated the proportion of health (mortality and morbidity) that may be accounted for by biological in contrast to social, environmental, and behavioral factors, with the latter factors carrying the most weight (ranging from 50% to 80% of the explanation of health outcomes; see McGinnis & Foege, 1993).

Theories of the Life Course

Whereas the early social and behavioral work focused on individual aging and the factors in successful aging, life satisfaction, adaptation, disengagement, and adjustment with advancing years, more recent studies focus on understanding the process of aging from the perspective of the life course and the relation of coping, social support, personal control, self-efficacy, and focus on the behavioral dimensions of aging. Here, aging individuals and cohorts are examined as one phase of the entire lifetime and seen as shaped by historical, social, economic, and environmental factors that occur at earlier lifecourse ages (Bengtson & Allen, 1993; George, 1993). In the work of George (1990) and others, life course theory bridges macro- and microlevels of analysis by considering the relationships between social structure, social processes, and social psychological states. Nevertheless, the primary focus is more on the microlevel, with an emphasis on how macrolevel phenomena influence *individuals.* In a recent review of these theories, Dannefer and Uhlenberg (1999) point to "three significant intellectual problems in theorizing about the life course: (a) a tendency to equate the significance of social forces with social change, (b) a neglect of intracohort variability, and (c) an unwarranted affirmation of choice as an unproblematized determinant of the life course" (p. 309). Insofar as theories of personality and the aging process seek explanations at the individual level, these theories are of limited utility in explaining how public policies of the state, the economic system, the sex/gender system, and the medical-industrial complex influence health and aging in society (Estes, Gerard, & Clarke, 1984).

Social Constructionist Theories

Another set of theories at the microlevel, but linked to the macrolevel through processes of social interaction, is characterized by social constructionism (Estes, 1979; Gubrium & Holstein, 1999). In the earliest development of a political economy theory of aging, Estes (1979) begins with this proposition:

> The major problems faced by the elderly in the United States are, in large measure, ones that are socially constructed as a result of our conceptions of aging and the aged. What is done for and about the elderly, as well as what we know about them, including knowledge gained from research, are products of our conceptions of aging. In an important sense, then, the major problems faced by the elderly are the ones we create for them. (p. 1)

Later, Estes and her colleagues note, "A cornerstone of the political economy of public policy and aging . . . is the social construction of problems and the remedies to deal with them" (Estes, Linkins, & Binney, 1996, p. 349). As used with the political economy perspective, the constructed "problems" of aging and their policy remedies are examined in relation to (a) the capacity of strategically located agents and interests to define "the problem" and to press their views into public consciousness and law and (b) the objective facts of the situation (Estes, 1979).

Symbolic interactionist theories (Gubrium, 1967; Rose, 1967) posit that the interactional context and process (environment, persons, and encounters in it) may significantly affect the kind of aging process a person experiences. "Both self and society are seen as capable of creating new alternatives" (Estes, 1979). The social construction of reality perspective provides several useful insights:

> The experience of old age is dependent in large part upon how others react to the aged; that is, social context and cultural meanings are important. Meanings are crucial in influencing how growing old is experienced by the aging in any given society; these meanings are shaped through interaction of the aged with the individuals, organizations, and institutions that comprise the social context. Social context, however, incorporates not only situational events and interactional opportunities but also structural constraints that limit the range of possible interaction and the degree of understanding, reinforcing certain lines of action while barring others. (Estes, 1981, p. 400)

Age Stratification and the Aging and Society Paradigm

Two macrolevel gerontological theories are age stratification (Riley, Johnson, & Foner, 1972) and its successor, the aging and society paradigm (Riley, Foner, & Riley, 1999). Age stratification attends to the role and influence of social structures on the process of individual aging and the stratification of age in society (Riley, 1998; Riley & Riley, 1994a, 1994b). This perspective looks at the differential experiences of age cohorts across time, as well as what Riley and Riley (1994a, 1994b) call the interdependence of changes in lives and changes in social structures.

A more recent dimension of this theory is the concept of structural lag, wherein social structures (e.g., policies of retirement at age 65) do not keep pace with changes in population dynamics and individual lives (such as increasing life expectancy). The age stratification approach is limited by a relative inattention to issues of power and social class relationships, especially insofar as these influence the social structure and the policies constituted by it, and ultimately to the experience of aging (Estes, Gerard, & Clarke, 1984). Quadagno and Reid (1999) summarize the criticisms that the theory "relied on an inherently static concept of social structure, that it neglected political processes inherent in the creation of inequality, and that it ignored institutionalized patterns of inequality" (p. 347).

In developing the *aging and society paradigm*, Matilda Riley and her colleagues (1999) addressed the "unintentionally static overtones of age stratification" by introducing "two dynamisms—changing lives and changing structures—as interdependent but distinct sets of processes" (p. 333), in which there is an interplay between them. In the tradition of functionalist theorizing, the emphasis is on social homeo-stasis (and imbalances), age integration, and the formation of norms. Although devoted to "describing and understanding age, as age affects individuals and also is embedded in and influences social structures" (Riley et al., 1999, p. 341), it flows out of the *consensus* rather than the *conflict* approach. It is the conflict approach on which the critical perspective proposed in this volume rests.

Critical Perspectives on Aging and Health

Critical perspectives emerged in response to the limitations of tradi-tional theorizing of aging. Critical analysis of traditional aging theories reveals how these theories avoid questioning the very social problems and conditions facing the elderly (Estes, 1979) and, therefore, have the tendency to reproduce rather than alter the conditions of the elderly. At a basic level, theories such as disengagement and activity can be seen as reinforcing ageist attitudes about the elderly and legitimating policies that reinforce dependency at the expense of empowerment. In addition, the association of age with disease and inevitable decline is better reframed so that aging is seen as a *social* rather than *biological process*. This alternative view of aging is central to the critical perspective be-cause many experiences related to aging result from socioeconomic conditions and inequalities experienced (and compounded) over the life course.

In attempting to bridge some of the issues of concern regarding the aforementioned aging theories—namely, fragmentation and the macro-micro problem—the critical approach proposed in this volume considers the multilevel relationships between social structure, social processes, and the population (Bengtson & Schaie, 1999; Estes et al., 1996). As applied within the political economy framework, the recur-sive relationship among levels of analysis is emphasized (Giddens, 1984), providing an avenue for extending and further synthesizing this micro-macro linkage. As such, issues of aging are not perceived as beginning with the individual, the generation, institutions or organi-zations, or society. Rather, all levels are viewed in terms of mutual dependency rather than opposition.

Although the field of critical approaches to social policy and aging has grown over the past decade, the promise of the field—namely, its incorporation of a variety of disciplinary perspectives—also contributes to the difficulty that the field faces in realizing its potential. As both Baars (1991) and Phillipson (1998) note, critical health and aging is a very broad field concerned primarily with questions and analyses that fall outside the mainstream of gerontology and other disciplines in the social sciences. These range from examining the role of the state and capital in managing the aging process (e.g., Estes, 1991a; Walker, 1999) to questions regarding the meaning and purpose of aging in the context of postmodern societies (Cole, 1992; Gubrium & Holstein, 1999). The critical perspective presented in this book seeks to address such questions.

The Critical Perspective:
A Theoretical Retrospective—1960s to the Present

The attraction of a broader critical perspective for younger scholars is at least partially attributable to activist scholars in the 1960s who became dissatisfied with the fragmented worldview of the separate and balkanized disciplines of political science, anthropology, sociology, history, and economics that failed to anticipate or explain the revolutionary social changes of the 1960s civil rights, peace, and women's movements (Gouldner, 1973). The distinct and largely historical disciplinary approaches of sociology and political science, for example, were clearly inadequate to deal with the growing complexity of social problems. The narrow conceptions of politics and government in political science (Stone & Harpham, 1982) and of the structural functionalist theories of the political and social order in sociology became the object of critical examination (Gouldner, 1970, 1973). In addition, the limits of the traditional social science approaches themselves were subject to criticism and became the major topic of study.

A blossoming literature in the sociology of knowledge raised serious questions about the possibility of a value-free social science, the problem of objectivity, and the ideological commitments inherent in positivist social science (Gouldner, 1973; Habermas, 1984). Also evolving was a feminist critique of the epistemological foundations of the dominant methodological and theoretical approaches in these disciplines (Smith, 1990). These strains and tensions opened social sciences further to interpretive and critical approaches.

Sweeping political and social changes during the 1960s were accompanied not only by students questioning authority but also by an explosion of theoretical and philosophical work challenging the "received" authority of the traditional disciplines and methodologies. These developments heightened the receptivity of U.S. scholars to the Frankfurt School's critique of "objective" positivist science as well as their receptivity to the Frankfurt School's commitment to the close relationship between theory and practice and the juncture between the academy and social action. This is called the theory-praxis relationship.

The rapidity, magnitude, and complexity of change, technology, and modernity, coupled with the increasing globalization of society and the growing awareness of the interconnectedness of the different spheres and sectors of society and the world have enlarged the scope of the work required to understand and resolve societal problems. There was dissatisfaction with behaviorism (focused on the behavior of individual actors) in political science that "was perceived as seriously restricting the problems one could investigate in a scientific manner . . . [and] inadequate to address such important issues as problems of equality and redistribution among classes, factions, and groups, the nature of justice and legitimacy, and the viability of democracy" (Stone & Harpham, 1982, p. 15).

All of these trends converged to elevate the significance and importance of the study of the role of intellectuals in the production of social thought, as well as the conduct of research at the macrohistorical and institutional level, however difficult. This was accompanied by growing interest in the potentially emancipatory and empowering role of knowledge (see Habermas, 1971), which speaks to the generative relation of the subject to the world. These influences have been joined by the interest in modernism and postmodernism and the formal linguistic self-consciousness that has transformed the notion of "culture" and that foregrounds issues of language and promotes a broad interest in culture, symbolic forms, communication, and meaning.

The emergence of logical positivism (with its emphasis on language and knowledge) and phenomenology (emphasizing meaning and consciousness) has led to new formulations of a "critical humanism" from a broad range of theorists, including Lukacs, Korsch, and the Frankfurt School; Brecht and Benjamin (influenced by artistic movements); and Gramsci and Lefebvre (emphasizing the need for historical and social specificity) (Arato & Gebhardt, 1982). Of particular note is the focus on the creation of meaningful social realities and on culture and ideology as the site of both domination and resistance. The critical analysis of popular culture is deemed as crucial for any political strategy because, as Gramsci and others have argued, ideas can have the weight of material force.

The experience and failures of the Frankfurt School illustrate the difficulties in conceptualizing and implementing an agenda of research in the critical and political economy theory of aging (Arato & Gebhardt, 1982). It requires an openly critical, reflexive, and interdisciplinary approach that flies in the face of the current organizational structure of, and advancement within, the social science disciplines. The social and political risks to scholars who cut cross-lots in the academy and elsewhere, coupled with the pressures for immediate (instrumental) answers from those working in policy fields, work against the integration of theoretical and methodological work that was first envisioned by the Frankfurt School.

Major Theoretical Perspectives in the Critical Approach

Critical approaches to social policy and aging build on an array of intellectual traditions, including the works of Karl Marx, Max Weber, Antonio Gramsci, the Frankfurt School and more recently Jürgen Habermas, state theorists such as Claus Offe and James O'Connor, psychoanalytic perspectives (Biggs, 1997), and the contemporary work of Anthony Giddens. Using this theoretical seedbed, a field of critical gerontology has emerged and coalesced over the past decade with work in the United States and Europe. Four broad theoretical areas constitute and inform the field of political economy: conflict, critical, feminist, and cultural. Scholars writing from any one of these theoretical domains may draw on the others in pursuing their work (see Figure 2.1).

Conflict Theories

Those working from a *conflict theoretical approach* contend that society and its social order are held together by the dominance of certain groups and structural interests over others. The outcomes of conflict and power struggles are posited as explanations of how society is organized and how it functions, and society is seen as held together

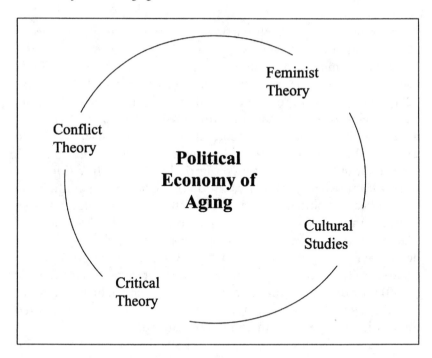

Figure 2.1. Theoretical Roots of Political Economy of Aging

by constraint rather than by consensus (Collins, 1988). It is argued that societal institutions such as work organizations and medicine are organized the way they are and operate the ways they do because some manage to successfully impose their ideas, material interests, and actions on others. Not only is conflict theory about social change, it

> concerns explaining social stability as a general theory of society. But it differs from functionalist theory in seeing social order as the product of contending interests and the resources groups have for dominating one another and negotiating alliances and coalitions. Its basic focus . . . [is] (in Dahrendorf's terms) latent conflict; it deals with social order as domination and negotiation. . . . Conflict theory is not surprised by . . . upheavals and changes . . . war or revolution. . . . It sees social order as maintained by forces of domination that cling to the status quo and attempt to legitimate it by traditional ideals; but leaves tremendous stores of social energy locked up in latent opposition, capable of being suddenly released by a catalytic event. (Collins, 1988, p. 118)

The state not only actively participates in these struggles but also reflects various forms of the interests to the most powerful. A variety of neo-Marxist (O'Connor, 1973; Offe & Keane, 1984), neo-Weberian (Alford & Friedland, 1985; Habermas, 1975), and neo-Gramscian theories (Hall, 1996; Sassoon, 1987a) of the state fall within this perspective. A contrasting view of society emerges from the *social order theoretical approach*, built on consensus theories that posit that society is held together by shared values and broad agreement across different groups in society about the way society is organized and how it functions (Parsons, 1951). Two major theories within the social order paradigm, liberal political and pluralist theories, portray the state as a neutral entity, operating in the universal interest of all members of society (Estes, Gerard, & Clarke, 1984). Critics of the social order paradigm fault it for idealizing democracy and "public choice" while overlooking the power of big, economically concentrated, and dominant interests. Schattschneider (1960) introduced the concept of the "mobilization of bias" to describe how these powerful dominant interests are built into (i.e., structured) the way interest group politics and the state operate.

Critical Theories

Critical theory is "designed with a practical intent, to criticize and subvert domination in all its forms" (Bottomore, 1983, p. 183). It is a critical perspective on all social practices [that is] . . . preoccupied by a critique of ideology—of systematically distorted accounts of reality which attempt to conceal and legitimate asymmetrical power relations . . . [and how] social interests, conflicts and contradictions are expressed in thought, and how they are produced and reproduced in systems of domination . . . to enhance awareness of the roots of domination, undermine ideologies and help to compel changes in consciousness and action. (Bottomore, 1983, p. 183)

The work of Antonio Gramsci is particularly relevant in three regards: his work on (a) the theory of ideological hegemony (ruling or dominant ideas of the period), (b) the role of intellectuals, and (c) the "theory of praxis" in which thought and action (research and policy or practice) are linked. Often described as a member of the Frankfurt School, Gramsci was concerned with the divergence between people's ideas and their economic conditions. He argued that a critical examination of popular culture and beliefs was crucial and that ideas can have the weight of material (economic) force.

Feminist Theories

Another set of theories constituting the critical approach to social policy and aging are feminist theories. Feminist theories, which are complementary and often related to or included in the political economy perspective, emphasize the importance of gender by examining the gender biases in social science research and the production of knowledge and practice. Gender is a crucial organizing principle in the economic and power relations of societal institutions as well as of social life throughout the life course. Gender therefore influences and shapes the experience of aging (Calasanti, 1993; Calasanti & Zajicek, 1993; Diamond, 1992; Estes, 1998b; Ginn & Arber, 1995; McMullin, 1995) and the distribution of resources in old age to men and women.

In the United States, feminist theorists have attended to the state (Acker, 1988; MacKinnon, 1989; Orloff, 1993) but, with a few exceptions (Calasanti, 1996; Calasanti & Zajicek, 1993; Estes & Binney, 1990; Harrington Meyer, 1990, 1996; Quadagno, 1988), have not generally focused on old age. There is little consensus on the paradigm of feminist theory of the state, and the political spectrum has been debated from the "right" to the "left." Chafetz (1997) speaks of the "normative emphasis" in the focus on gender studies and defines feminist theory to include the following:

1. Normative discussions of how societies and relations ought to be structured, their current inequalities, and strategies to achieve equity
2. Critiques of androcentric classical theories, concepts, epistemologies, and assumptions
3. Explanatory theories of the relation of gender and social, cultural, economic, psychological, and political structures and processes

Catherine MacKinnon (1989) points out the strength of a critical and Marxist perspective as a "point of departure" for theorizing about women and the state:

Marxism is . . . the contemporary theoretical tradition that—whatever its limitations—confronts organized social dominance, analyzes it in dynamic rather than static terms, identifies social forces that systematically shape social imperatives, and seeks to explain human freedom both within and against history. It confronts class, which is real. It offers both a critique of the inevitability and inner coherence of social injustice and a theory of the necessity and possibilities of change. (p. ix)

Gayle Rubin (1975) contends that Marxian analysis is important for feminist work because it is consistent with the perspective that the sex/gender system is the product of historical human activity. As discussed in Chapter 1, the sex/gender system is a set of arrangements by which a society transforms biological sexuality into products of human activity.

Several key concepts must be incorporated in any serious feminist theory of the state and old age. Important analytic work addresses (a) the two tiers of social policy: social assistance and social insurance; (b) the concepts of the gendered wage and the family wage; and (c) the understanding of how older women's fate in the welfare state is based on her marital status and her husband's work history and how the concept of the traditional autonomous nuclear family is inculcated into law and social policy. Significant work is needed on the various processes of social control inculcated in the state and society that confront women across the life course and their effects on the life situation of old women. Joan Acker's (1988, 1992) concept of "gendered institutions" as applied to the state is extremely useful for a feminist approach to old age. She contributes the significant idea that there are two key social processes of the state: the *relations of distribution* and the *relations of production*. Fruitful topics of research from the feminist perspective on aging in the United States are the specification of gendered policy, the processes and structures in and through which policy operates, and the gendered outcomes.

Cultural Studies

Cultural studies are "a dissenting movement" that "helps to understand the mechanisms of cultural power . . . and the means to resist them" (Sardar & Van Loon, 1997, pp. 170-171). Three noteworthy characteristics of cultural study are that it

[1] aims to examine its subject matter in terms of *cultural practices* and their *relation to power*. Its constant goal is to expose power relationships and

examine how these relationships influence and shape cultural practices ... ; [2] [seeks] to analyze the *social and political context* within which (culture) manifests itself ... [and] [3] is committed to a *moral evaluation* of modern society and to a *radical line of political action.* The tradition of cultural studies is not one of value free scholarship, but one committed to social reconstruction by critical political involvement. Thus cultural studies aims to *understand and change structures* of dominance everywhere, but in industrial capitalist societies in particular. (Sardar & Van Loon, 1997, pp. 8-9; italics in original)

Clearly, within the cultural studies tradition, there are differing, if not a dizzying number of, theoretical and methodological perspectives and emphases, including those that consider ideological hegemony as a cultural element that "binds society together without the use of force" (Sardar & Van Loon, 1997, p. 49). For Gramsci, culture is a key site where struggles for hegemony take place. For Hoggart, the dominant elite express power by projecting their "fields of value" as they accord legitimacy and exposure to their cultural forms and practices (Sardar & Van Loon, 1997).

Cultural studies have contributed a political dimension and the study of such fields of value. This work is potentially *empowering* and *emancipating* "by encouraging . . . [people] with the resources to understand the intrinsic relationship between culture and the various forms of power, and thus to develop strategies for survival" (Sardar & Van Loon, 1997, p. 43). With such knowledge among the people, the potentially revolutionary human subject may act.

Applying the Critical Theoretical Approach to Aging

A central and unifying tenet among these theories is the notion that aging and the problems faced by the elderly are socially constructed and result from societal conceptions of aging and the aged (Estes, 1979). This process occurs at both the macrolevel and microlevel as well as at the mesolevel of organizations that operate between the microlevel and the macrolevel. The state and economy (macrolevel) can be seen as influencing the experience and condition of aging, but individuals also actively construct their worlds through personal inter-actions (microlevel) and through organizational and institutional structures and processes (mesolevel) that constitute their social worlds and society.

The Political Economy of Aging

The political economy of aging offers an important approach to understanding the condition and experience of social policy and aging drawing from multiple theories and levels of analysis (see Table 2.1). Beginning in the late 1970s and early 1980s with the work of Estes (1979), Guillemard (1980), Phillipson (1982), and Walker (1981), these theorists initiated the task of describing the role of capitalism and the state in contributing to systems of domination and marginalization of the aged. On the basis of the continuing work of these and other authors developing a critical perspective on theories of aging (Marshall & Tindale, 1978) and theories of the welfare state (Myles, 1984; Quadagno, 1988), the political economy perspective is classified as one of the major theories in social gerontology (Bengtson et al., 1997; Bengtson & Schaie, 1999; Hendricks & Leedham, 1991; Marshall, 1996; Phillipson, 1999; Walker, 1999). The political economy perspective is distinguished from the dominant liberal-pluralist theory in political science and sociology by according greater importance to the economic system and other social structures and forces in shaping and reproducing the prevailing power structure of society. In the political economy perspective, social policies pertaining to retirement income, health, and social service benefits and entitlements are seen as products of economic, political, and sociocultural processes and forces that interact in any given sociohistorical period (Estes, 1991a, 2000a). Social policy is an outcome of the social struggles, conflicts, and dominant power relations of the period. Policy reflects the structure and culture of advantage and disadvantage as enacted through class, race/ethnicity, gender, and age relations. Concurrently, social policy stimulates power struggles along these structural lines of class, race/ethnicity, gender, and age. Social policy is itself a powerful determinant of the life chances and conditions of individuals and population groups such as the elderly.

As noted in Chapter 1, a central assumption of the political economy perspective is that the phenomena of aging and old age are directly related to the nature of the society in which they are situated. Therefore, they cannot be considered or analyzed in isolation from other societal forces and phenomena. The power of the state, business, and labor and

Table 2.1   Theoretical Contributions to the Political Economy of Aging: Estes Version

Microlevel Theories	Mesolevel Theories	Macrolevel Theories
Symbolic interaction	Organizational	Conflict
Social constructionism		Political economy
Labeling		Critical
Cultural studies		Sociology of knowledge
		Feminist
	Linking Theories	
	Cultural studies	
	Political economy	
	Critical	
	Feminist	
	Interactionist	
	Sociology of knowledge	

SOURCE: Adapted from Marshall (1996).

the role of the economy are central concerns. Explicitly recognized in this framework are the structural influences on the aging experience, including the role of societal institutions and social relations in understanding how aging and old age are defined and treated in society and the role of ideology in shaping those definitions and policy options for their treatment. The major problems facing the elderly, such as dependency, are understood as socially constructed and a result of societal conceptions of aging and the aged (Estes, 1979). As Estes and her colleagues describe it,

> The significance of the political economy literature is in its directing attention to how the treatment of older people in society and the experience of old age itself are related to an economy whose boundaries are no longer limited to the U.S. alone but include worldwide economic and political conditions.... The task of the political economy of aging is to locate society's treatment of the aged in the context of the economy (national and international), the role of the state, the conditions of the labor market, and the class, sex, race, ethnic, and age divisions in society. This will require serious consideration of the relationship of capitalism to aging. (Estes, Gerard, & Clarke, 1984, pp. 11-12)

Moral Economy and Humanistic Gerontology

The development of cultural and humanistic gerontology, sometimes referred to as moral economy, is best understood in the context of the larger field of cultural studies. The development of moral economy is part of a broad field of *cultural gerontology*. This approach has gained popularity, as the classical theoretical opposition of structure *versus* agency and culture *versus* structure has given way to an appreciation of the interplay and "recursive" relationships of culture, structure, and agency (Estes, 1999a; Giddens, 1991). Cultural gerontology is part of the trend toward theories that reject the sole determinacy of economics in explaining social institutions such as the state and old age policy. There has been a reformulation of the unidirectional causality implied in the classical "base superstructure" model of Marxism. What has followed is an intensified focus on questions of meaning and experience.

Humanistic gerontology adds still another dimension to critical approaches to health and aging, by seeking both to critique existing theories and to construct new positive models of aging based on research by historians, ethicists, and social scientists (Bengtson, Burgess, & Parrott, 1997; Cole, Achenbaum, Jakobi, & Kastenbaum, 1993). Moody (1993b) identifies several goals for the critical humanistic perspective in gerontology, including (a) developing theories that emphasize and reveal the subjective and interpretive dimensions of aging, (b) commitment to praxis and social change, and (c) the production of emancipatory knowledge. Consistent with and complementary to both the political economy and feminist theories, this approach centers on the concepts and relations of power, social action, and social meanings as they pertain to aging. At the core, this approach is concerned with the absence of meaning in the lives of the elderly and the sense of doubt and uncertainty that is thought to permeate and influence their day-to-day lives and social relations (Moody, 1988a, 1988b, 1997).

In the United States, theories of moral economy have developed largely as part of the political economy of aging (Minkler & Cole, 1991, 1999; Minkler & Estes, 1991, 1999). Building on the work of E. P. Thompson (1963), Kohli (1987), Minkler and Cole (1991), and others, those working from a moral economy perspective in gerontology have brought attention to the social norms and reciprocal obligations and relations and their role in the social integration and social control of the elderly and the workforce, among other concerns. U.S. proponents of this perspective are Hendricks and Leedham (1991), Minkler and Cole (1991, 1999), Moody (1988b, 2000), Robertson (1999), and others. The concept of moral economy reflects popular consensus concerning the legitimacy of certain practices based on shared views of social norms and obligations (Robertson, 1999, p. 39). Scholars working from the moral economy perspectives attend to issues of distributive and economic justice and norms such as reciprocity and generational equity.

The cultural and symbolic elements incorporated under cultural gerontology necessarily include the ideas, beliefs, ideologies, norms, and meanings that are an essential part of the construction of old age and old age policy. The institutions of work, retirement, the family, and the state both *reflect* and *affect* these symbolic and cultural elements. These symbolic and cultural elements are and have always been an essential part of the constructionist perspective on aging that Estes (1972) first proposed and later joined with a political economy analysis in *The Aging Enterprise* (Estes, 1979).

Because thinking about cultural sociology and postmodernism is often cast in oppositional terms to the determinacy of economics as the engines of state policy, it is important to clarify the place of culture in the political economy framework developed here.

Ideology

Consciousness is culture. Ideology is culture. It is noteworthy that "culture is anything but neutral" (Parenti, 1999, p. 11). An examination of ideology is an essential element of any work under the rubric of moral or political economy. Intellectual arguments and theoretical oppositions are likely to be about the following: (a) whether one subscribes to a determinacy for the cultural concepts of ideology and/or social norms in producing state policy on aging (and the institution of retirement, etc.)—for example, whether one argues that ideology determines or is merely part of a larger array of influencing factors that shape state policy—and (b) the processes by which phenomena (such as ideology or norms) develop and have their influence. The issue is whether ideology and norms emerge through coercive processes of social struggle and conflict *versus* processes of consensual agreement in society concerning values and norms.

The view advanced here is that (a) ideology is an essential (but not the only) element in the framing of state and social action that culminates in social policy on aging and (b) the consent of the governed occurs through struggle—political, material, and ideological. Cultural products are contested, emerging, evolving, and problematic. Nevertheless, we must always account for the recursive relations of agency, culture, and structure (Giddens, 1991).

Work in the political economy of aging (Estes, 1991a, 1999a) deals extensively with the power struggles over ideology and over the legitimacy of both state actions and the state itself. To say it another way for emphasis, legitimating and delegitimating ideologies and practices are cultural products and ones over which there are enormous struggles. As such, ideology and other cultural phenomena are both the "object of study" and the "location of political criticism and action," consistent with substantial work in what is now called cultural studies (Sardar & Van Loon, 1997).

Conclusion

A critical perspective on social policy and aging provides the tools to understand the broad social, economic, and political factors and structural arrangements that are integral to and that produce old age. It provides a direct challenge to the dominant and mainstream thinking in gerontology that tends to reduce aging to an individual problem of dependency. This chapter discusses the limitations of the prevailing gerontological theories and provides an alternative critical approach. The theoretical roots of the critical perspective— (a) conflict theories, (b) critical theories, (c) feminist theories, and (d) cultural studies— are presented to understand the application of a critical political economy theoretical approach. Application to fields of gerontology study (e.g., the moral economy and humanistic gerontology) is made, and the importance of ideology is elucidated.

3

The Medicalization and Commodification of Aging and the Privatization and Rationalization of Old Age Policy

Carroll L. Estes
Steven P. Wallace
Karen W. Linkins
Elizabeth A. Binney

Old age, aging, and the policies designed for the elderly in the United States are profoundly shaped by four social processes: (a) the biomedicalization of aging, (b) the commodification of aging, (c) the privatization of old age policy, and (d) the rationalization of old age policy. This chapter describes these processes and examines their consequences for the older persons in America.

AUTHORS' NOTE: Some material in this chapter is adapted from "Political Economy of Health and Aging," by C. L. Estes, S. P. Wallace, and K. W. Linkins. In *Handbook of Medical Sociology* (5th ed.), edited by C. E. Bird, P. Conrad, and A. M. Fremont (pp. 129-142). (Upper Saddle River, NJ: Prentice Hall, 2000).

The Biomedicalization of Aging

With the substantial reduction in deaths from acute illnesses during the past century, mortality has shifted largely to the chronic conditions most common in "old age." This concentration of disease at advanced ages has coincided with the substantial increase in the social and technical power of the medical profession, setting the stage for the dominance of biomedicine and its way of viewing life over old age.

As a discipline and a "worldview," medicine has been one of the most important and powerful forces in the 20th century. As a paradigm, the biomedical model focuses on individual organic pathology, physiological etiologies, and biomedical interventions. This approach has tremendous political consequences, as Conrad and Schneider (1992) attest: "The medical profession . . . has a virtual monopoly over anything that is defined as illness or a 'medical treatment' " (p. 36). Estes and Binney (1989) note that two dimensions of the biomedicalization of aging are key: first, the social construction of aging as a medical problem—that is, thinking of aging itself primarily as a disease and/or medical problem as defined by medical practitioners—and, second, the praxis (or practice) of aging as a medical problem and the behaviors and policies growing out of thinking of aging in this way.

The biomedical model emphasizes the etiology, clinical treatment, and management of diseases of the elderly as defined and treated by medical practitioners, while giving marginal attention to the social and behavioral processes and problems of aging. As the primary "institutionalized thought structure" (Berger & Luckmann, 1966) of the field of aging, the model influences everything else—research and the development of knowledge in the field, gerontological and geriatric practice, policy making, and public perceptions. The equation of old age with illness has encouraged society to think about old age as a pathological, abnormal, and an undesirable state, which in turn shapes the attitudes of members of society toward the elderly and of the elderly toward themselves (Estes, 1979). Sick role expectations (Parsons, 1951) may result in behaviors such as social withdrawal; reduction of activity; increased dependency (Arluke & Peterson, 1981; Townsend, 1981); and the loss of self-esteem, efficacy, and personal sense of control (Rodin & Langer, 1977)—all of which increase the social control of the elderly through medical definition and management (Estes & Binney, 1989; Estes, Gerard, Zones, & Swan, 1984).

The dominance of the medical model in aging obscures the extent to which illness and other problems of the elderly are influenced or determined by potentially modifiable social factors, such as (a) income and education, (b) safe and supportive housing environments that promote healthy behaviors, (c) opportunities for meaningful human connections, and (d) public financing for rehabilitation. In the 1970s, countermovements emerged in opposition to the medical dominance of health care for older persons. Home health care, provided largely through quasi-public nonprofit visiting nurses associations, grew in popularity as a way to assist persons who had left the hospital but needed ongoing professional services. Hospice care also evolved out of a social movement to demedicalize death and was built on the volunteer labor of laypersons in their own homes and communities (Abel, 1986). The net effect of both trends was to shift a significant amount of medical care out of the hospital and away from physicians into the home. Both trends also disproportionately affected the elderly and shifted substantial work from formal (paid) delivery systems to informal (unpaid) systems and, thus, predominantly onto women. By the end of the 1980s, however, financing of this care, especially through Medicare, brought medical oversight and control to these new services, even though the provision of care had been effectively transferred from the hospital to the home.

Despite the reality that the greatest burden of disease in old age now stems from chronic rather than acute conditions, public policy regarding medical care for the elderly clings to a medical engineering model, which constructs health and illness based on a rational system of causes within the context of the body's cellular and biochemical systems (Renaud, 1975). This model implies that it requires an expert (such as a physician) to fix problems, usually after they occur. This model also supports society's growing investment in medical care and technology as the primary determinant of good health (McKeown, 1978), despite the growing body of research that substantiates the significant effect on health in old age of behavior, environment, social inequalities, and other factors. One result of the dominance of this model is that federal research funding tends to follow dread diseases (breast cancer, Alzheimer's, etc.) on the assumption that an individual-level cure can be found.

The strength of the medical engineering model persists and grows in the new millennium as exemplified in *Science* magazine's claim that the scientific revolution in genetics and biology is likely to resolve the multiple problems of the entire U.S. economy as well as the demographics of aging. Pardes et al. (1999) contend that the human genome project and other scientific advances will solve the problems of both health and the costs of medical care—thereby solving the problems of the economy. The authors challenge the widely held belief among health economists that medical research, genetics, and technology actually generate higher, rather than lower, overall medical costs. Pardes et al. (1999) unabashedly argue in favor of greatly augmented state investments in biotechnology through the National Institutes of Health (NIH) because this investment will purportedly resolve many of the nation's economic, demographic, and health woes. They do not discuss how biomedical research will understand, address, and remedy the social, economic, and environmental elements (what sociologists call "root causes") such as economic and educational inequality. These elements are well documented as producing adverse health consequences at all ages and increasing both medical and societal costs.

Critics of the biomedical model point to the proclivity of this approach toward individualistic and reductionist thinking and to erroneously equating (and conflating) the needs and definitions of physicians and the medical profession with the needs of the society—and in this case, the needs of the aging and an aging society (Estes & Binney, 1989). A leading critic of biomedicalization, Ivan Illich (1976) in *Medical Nemesis,* introduced and applied the concept of "social iatrogenesis" (the medical creation of illness) to the outcomes of medical care. He argues that medicine is more a *threat* to health than it is a healing force. Illich even proposes that medicine be dismantled and replaced by different forms of self-help.

The power of the medical model has drained resources for the scholarship necessary to pursue promising alternative social, behavioral, and environmental approaches, while simultaneously encouraging the all-American "magic bullet" mentality for those seeking the "nirvana" of a happy and eternal life. Although biomedicine merits a respected place for its contributions to social policy and aging, its extension to and control over all aspects of life diminish its own effectiveness and divert the field from the essential and critical work needed to understand the complex social and environmental factors that significantly shape, structure, and modify the basic processes of old age and aging on multiple levels.

The Commodification of Old Age and the Privatization of Medical Care

Commodification of Old Age

Commodification is the process of taking a good or service that has been produced and used, but not bought or sold, and turning it into an item that is exchanged for money. The continuing and growing influence of the medical engineering model of health has contributed to the commodification of old age and aging over the past century (Estes, 1979). This is reflected in the shift in the mode of production of medical goods and services from an orientation of fulfilling human needs (such as food, shelter, or functional assistance for the disabled) to a mode of medical production oriented toward monetary exchange for the creation of private profit and increasingly enormous private wealth. Commodification diminishes the consideration of social needs and the "right" of the elderly to health and health care (Caplan, Light, & Daniels, 1999; Estes & Binney, 1989; Estes, Gerard, Zones, et al., 1984). Although helping an ill loved one bathe and dress does not involve a commodity relationship, hiring a personal care worker to do those same tasks commodifies it. Medicalization is involved because these new goods and services have been defined as medically related, and, therefore, medical providers serve as gatekeepers.

This view of care as a commodity is consistent with one of the central features of capitalism—that labor is treated as a commodity, being bought by business at the lowest possible price (Twine, 1994). This view resulted in the logical development of the concept of retirement when the changing methods of production in industry created the need for business (capital) to replace older and more expensive members of the labor force to maximize profits (Graebner, 1980). Creation of an age-defined end to employability along with the separation of the home from the workplace under capitalism were central forces in devaluing old age.

Although the commodification of labor is a hallmark of capitalist production, the growth imperative of capitalist systems also leads to the expansion of markets for existing products, and the creation of new products to sell. These products can be "new," or they can be products and services that had formerly been produced for immediate use (typically within the family) but now are produced for sale to others (such as prepared foods or caregiving services). In the United States, medical care for the elderly has long been a commodity. Within the capitalist system, there is an incentive to maximize profits rather than health, unless the level of health drags on productivity (Chernomas, 1999; Estes, Gerard, Zones, & Swan, 1984; Renaud, 1975). Despite an early tradition of charitable medical care, doctors and hospitals have always charged for their services (fee-for-service) when possible. Historically, hospitals were mostly stand-alone nonprofit facilities controlled primarily by doctors for whom these facilities were their personal workshops. Hospitals "sold" nonprofit medical care, but their institutional interests were less in profits and more in providing conditions desirable for physician practice and in creating community goodwill for financial donations and patient referrals.

The medical profession has been organized, historically, along a guild model with physician control over the education, licensing, and practice of medicine (Starr, 1982) and providing the basis of the legal right to practice through state law. Although interested in their own pecuniary benefit, doctors did not organize as other businesses along rational-bureaucratic lines. Since the 1980s and 1990s, corporate medicine has forced a degree of rationalization on the practice of medicine through the consolidation of medical industries and the growth of for-profit managed care. These latter trends raise controversial questions concerning whether doctors are becoming "proletarianized" as regular salaried workers—that is, employees who are forced to relinquish their positions of control and ownership of their own means of the production of medicine (Coburn, 1999; McKinlay & Stoeckle, 1988).

The first major boost to the commodification of health care in the United States occurred in 1946 with the passage of the Hill-Burton Law, which subsidized the private sector for construction and expansion of hospital facilities. With the passage of Medicare (medical services for the elderly) and Medicaid (medical care for the poor) in 1965, the long-term financial needs of the medical care industry were secured through the financial underwriting by the state of extravagantly technical and expensive medical centers (Estes, Gerard, Zones, & Swan, 1984). Hospitals and nursing homes were provided "cost-based" payments where allowable costs included the interest payments on new facilities and equipment as well as profits. These developments created a "gold rush" for the modern hospital and medical care, resulting in a "medical-industrial complex" (Ehrenreich & Ehrenreich, 1971; also see Chapter 8, "The Medical-Industrial Complex and the Aging Enterprise"). The Complex is composed of hospitals, drug companies, insurers, and suppliers with unknown billions of dollars in after-tax profits.

Government subsidies for the lucrative "American health empire" (Ehrenreich & Ehrenreich, 1971) have included tax deductions for employer-based health insurance, publicly funded health personnel training as well as hospital and nursing home construction, tax deductions for medical expenses, tax exemptions to nonprofit facilities, and substantial funding for the NIH in biological and biomedical research (in the multibillions annually and growing wildly, even during the budget deficit hysteria of the 1990s, the profits of which are later realized in the private market). For-profit hospital chains began to grow in prominence, expanding in suburban and Sunbelt areas where there was private insurance and little competition from or loyalty to nonprofit hospitals.

With Medicare and "cost-based" reimbursement, there was little risk involved and hospitals were guaranteed profits. For-profit nursing homes similarly grew in number dramatically during this time. Services were increasingly provided because of the revenues they generated, and there was increased concern over "provider-induced demand" for medical care. The net result was to reinforce an acute care model of medical services with a technological and institutional approach to the health care of older persons via the payment for hospital and physician services for elders under Medicare and for nursing home care for the poor elderly under Medicaid.

By the early days of the Reagan presidency, John Iglehart, editor of *Health Affairs,* observed, "Business and government have begun to look at medical care as more nearly an economic product than a social good" (Iglehart, 1982, p. 120). The transformation of the health needs of the aging into commodities for specific economic markets has helped produce the "aging enterprise" (Estes, 1979). This set of interests benefits from a definition of aging as a problem to be dealt with by experts. It supports a high-technology, pharmaceutically intensive, and specialized expert-led approach to treat parts of the problem presented by older "consumers" (more recently called "customers") who seek goods and services in the medical marketplace. (The aging enterprise is discussed in more detail in Chapter 8.) The concept of a "health care consumer" has been developed and refined as part of the

legitimating system of an individualistic, commodified form of medical care (e.g., consumer report cards for HMOs in the 1990s) (Estes,
Wallace, & Linkins, 2000).

Treating health care as a commodity for consumption shifts the
responsibility for many decisions that influence access, quality, and
cost to atomized individuals who, according to economic theory, make
theoretically available and rational "choices" in a market. This may be
contrasted with a "social rights" approach (Twine, 1994) that treats the
elderly and others as citizens with an entitlement to health care that is
ensured by the state and that is independent of their "property rights"
or ability to pay privately in the market (Myles, 1984).

Privatization

Although 40% of U.S. health care is financed by the federal government, these and other funds flow primarily to the private sector
medical-industrial complex, with the state limiting its own activities to
supporting and complementing the market (Estes, 1991a). For the elderly, the state role is primarily the public financing of health insurance
for the elderly and disabled (Medicare) and for the poor (Medicaid).
Furthering a process that began with the passage of Medicare and
Medicaid in 1965, the Reagan administration initiated policies that
dramatically fueled the growth in the for-profit service sector and in
overall U.S. health care costs (Fuchs, 1988). As a result of policies to
foster privatization and competition in medical care, the size of the
medical-industrial complex tripled during Reagan's presidential term
of office.

Through the regulation and financing of medical care and social
services, state policy under Reagan intensified the state's role in stimulating market investment opportunities for private capital (a form of
privatization). This occurred particularly in areas that traditionally
had been the domain of nonprofit health entities (Marmor, Schlesinger, &
Smithey, 1987) and that promised the greatest likelihood of profit
(e.g., hospital and home health services). State policy also increased
opportunities for private capital through civil law and regulation by
protecting the market and encouraging the participation of proprietary health entities (e.g., the Omnibus Reconciliation Act of 1980),
including the nearly $30 billion federal tax subsidy for the purchase
of private health insurance. President Reagan's additional public

subsidies in the form of tax cuts for capital, combined with the promotion of for-profit medical care, worked against one another in contradictory fashion to exacerbate the fiscal problems of the state (Estes, 1991b) by increasing the federal deficit.

Most recently, privatization has been proposed by a number of politicians as a way to theoretically improve the long-term financial health of Medicare. In 1999, a federal commission considered but failed to agree on a recommendation to shift Medicare to a "premium support" (also known as voucher) model (National Bipartisan Commission on the Future of Medicare, 1999). This would have provided private insurance companies a lucrative new market while reducing the social insurance features of Medicare and effectively reducing access to care by the elderly with the highest need and least money (Wallace, Enriquez-Haass, & Markides, 1998). Similar proposals were made by politicians in the 2000 presidential elections.

The increased privatization of virtually all aspects of medical care is the subject of controversy concerning the proper role of government. The extent of health services privatization depends, as Scarpaci (1989) notes, on the specific nature of conflict among capital, the state, the private sector, and health care consumers. A dominant and ideological view in the United States is that the market and business sectors can administer programs more efficiently than politicians and bureaucrats. Some public opinion polls even indicate that the public believes that the market system may be more fair than the political system (Lane, 1986).

Emerging through the processes of privatization is an altered form of the welfare state in which the context is shifted from the public sector role itself to a sector coordinating public-private linkages. The private sector, including the vast trillion-dollar U.S. medical-industrial complex, represents major stakeholders in this emerging new form. Social welfare expenditures, broadly defined with Social Security included, are relatively large expenditures at all levels of government. Privatization breaks the constraints on the use of public resources and puts them to multiple ends: to provide welfare and to secure profits (Nelson, 1995). The fundamental principle driving the development of the welfare state was for economic development to feed social development and, in so doing, to minimize inequality. Privatization, however, exemplifies an economic development strategy that is likely to escalate inequality (Chernomas, 1999).

A fundamental debate is whether privatization will actually lower (or increase) costs and improve efficiency in health care and long-term care, given the continuing pluralistic financing, complexity, and fragmentation of services, as well as the added costs of for-profit marketing, administration, and profit taking. Presently, there is little evidence that for-profit institutions and operating mechanisms will actually lower costs of health and long-term care. In fact, in Chile, where a significant part of the formerly universal public health insurance was privatized, costs and inefficiency have both increased (Larrañaga, 1999). The case that Bradford Gray made in the early 1990s about medical for-profit entities appears to still hold. Gray (1986) notes that there is little research to support the commonly held view that for-profit hospitals demonstrate lower costs or greater efficiency than do nonprofit facilities. Several more recent studies confirm "the high costs of investor owned care" and in particular that

> market medicine's dogma, that the profit motive optimizes care and minimizes costs, seems impervious to evidence that contradicts it. For decades, studies have shown that for-profit hospitals are 3 to 11% more expensive than not-for-profit hospitals [2,3,4,5,6,7]; no peer-reviewed study has found that for-profit hospitals are less expensive. For-profit hospitals spend less on personnel,[2,3,5,6] avoid providing charity care[4,8,9] and shorten stays. (Woolhandler & Himmelstein, 1999, p. 444)

There is a major debate about quality issues as well in nonprofit versus for-profit facilities. Two recent research studies from Harvard and Johns Hopkins Universities found disparities in the treatment of patients at for-profit dialysis centers, who are less likely to get transplants than those at nonprofit dialysis centers where improving the outcome of a client is more important than the loss of their business (Woolhandler & Himmelstein, 1999). This is consistent with findings of other research regarding the provision of home health care to the elderly that found poorer health outcomes for those served by for-profit health maintenance organizations (HMOs) than in fee for service (Shaughnessy, Schlenker, & Hittle, 1994). (The conversion of nonprofit to for-profit care is explored in greater detail in Chapter 4.)

In the 1980s, medical costs were rising rapidly and the U.S. economy experienced both inflation and recession, putting strong pressures on corporate profits. Rapidly rising medical costs exceeded the general rate of inflation many times and also generated pressures for cost containment and system rationalization. Relman (1980), editor of the *New England Journal of Medicine,* voiced the position of traditional craft-oriented physicians when he decried the "new medical-industrial complex" as shifting service delivery and control from nonprofit institutions and physicians to profit-making businesses. Corporate capital was expanding beyond the pharmaceutical and medical-device industries (where Relman felt it belonged), weakening the "best kind of regulation of the health care market place [which is] . . . the informed judgments of physicians working in the interests of their patients" (Relman, 1980, p. 967). The struggle by physicians to retain their medical dominance remains central and can be understood in a political economy framework that sees the transformation of medicine under capitalism through the phases of entrepreneurial, monopoly, and global capitalism (Coburn, 1999).

Throughout the 1980s and 1990s, there was a period of dramatic reorganization of American medicine toward a for-profit industrial model. Medicare legislation in the 1980s promoted for-profit entry into the medical field, including the shift toward for-profit home health care (Estes, Harrington, & Davis, 1992), the establishment of a new Medicare hospice benefit that helped eliminate its community-based voluntary organization (Abel, 1986), and the rationalization of hospital care through hospital reimbursement based on diagnosis rather than actual costs (Estes, Swan, & associates, 1993). As the for-profit sector grew in size and power, nonprofits were required by reimbursement and market practices to become part of chains and to operate increasingly like for-profits (Estes & Alford, 1990; also see Chapter 4). These practices by nonprofits, in turn, perversely contributed to a loss of legitimacy by nonprofit institutions (Estes, Binney, & Bergthold, 1989b). HMOs grew in popularity first with private employers and later with government as a way to contain costs. HMOs started primarily as nonprofit organizations but mostly changed to for-profit during the 1980s and 1990s to fund expansion and, coincidentally, provide large buyouts to many executives. Commodification and privatization also extended into the general health insurance industry. Blue Cross was established as a nonprofit organization by hospitals to guarantee their payment during the depression, and Blue Shield followed as a medically controlled payer of physician care (Stevens, 1983). Those nonprofits were slowly marginalized by for-profit insurance companies' entry into health insurance in the 1950s, the growing importance of public payers beginning in the 1960s, and corporate pressures for cost controls in the 1970s (Krause, 1996). The rupture was complete as Blue Cross and Blue Shield plans nationally converted to for-profit businesses in the 1990s along with many nonprofit hospitals.

The Rationalization of Medical Care

The rationalization of care refers to the implementation of organizational structures and processes designed to increase efficiency and reduce waste and costs. A concept made famous in Max Weber's (1946) classic studies of bureaucratization and rationalization, these processes are characteristic of new waves of industrialization and the development of capitalism over time.

In medical care, a major trend of organizational restructuring began in the 1980s, characterized by a rash of corporate mergers and consolidations that only intensified in number and magnitude throughout the 1990s. The restructuring of health care in the pursuit of rationalization increased as big business formed purchaser alliances such as the Washington Business Group on Health (Bergthold, 1990). These groups have advocated for health care to take a more businesslike approach as a way to reduce rising health care costs. The pressure on provider organizations to restrain costs has opened many insurance companies, HMOs, hospitals, physician management groups, and others to both vertical and horizontal mergers. Increasingly, the key contests have large corporate and government payers on one side pushing for cost control and large corporate providers on the other side trying to rationalize their operations to increase economic efficiency. Meanwhile, doctors have defensively tried to retain some autonomy and control over the practice of medicine while their control over the recruitment of patients, contract negotiations, and their own fees has decreased (McKinlay & Hafferty, 1993; McKinlay & Stoeckle, 1988).

For the elderly, Medicare policy has been an important instrument in furthering these processes of the medicalization and commodification of aging and the privatization and rationalization of medical care delivery throughout the 1980s and 1990s. This has been accomplished with significant and growing state subsidies for medical care for the

aged, accompanied by federal and state deregulation, cost containment, and the development and promotion of for-profit managed care
organizations. Examples of rationalization are Medicare cost containment through prospective payment, increased beneficiary premiums
and copayments, managed care, and benefit reductions in home care.
The least rationalized sector of medicine is the nursing home industry,
which is just now starting to rationalize its internal operations as well
as integrate into networks, alliances, and chains, partly in response to
the pressures of managed care. Many nonprofit nursing home administrators worry that they will be forced by the economic focus of
managed care to compromise their missions of providing quality care
(Wallace, Cohen, Schnelle, Kane, & Ouslander, 2000).

Implications

Although there are a number of exciting theoretical developments in
the field (Bengtson & Schaie, 1999; Phillipson, 1998), social gerontology is characterized by an abundance of studies that demonstrate
theory-less empiricism and a bias toward social engineering. Most of
the applied research on the demographics, health, health care, and
health economics of aging takes the existing system for granted. It does
not "problematize" or raise questions about, or measure the broad
effects and societal costs of, the surging for-profit and managed care
medical industries, pluralistic financing, and fragmented and inadequate systems of care for the elderly. Instead, the "research problems"
concerning both individual and societal aging, and concerning the
organization, delivery, and financing of medical care, are generally
defined as *technical* and capable of administrative correction under the
existing system. There is an unstated (and implicitly positive) assumption that the continued dominance of medicine and its powerful alliances with and within profit-making corporations and the scientific
disciplines of genetics and economics will somehow resolve the nation's
problems regarding health and health care in an aging society.

Technical and statistical developments include demographic,
econometric, and actuarial modeling. The availability of national data
permits the production of what appear to be objective and precise
value-neutral calculations of the cost-benefits of health policy changes
but that embed a series of assumptions that work against the interests

of the elderly and much of society (Ubel, DeKay, Baron, & Asch, 1996). Such calculations are usually without consideration of the full array of *social costs* shifted onto others in society as shown by two examples:

1. The substantial cost of women's unpaid labor as their informal caring work has been increased with medical cost containment and technology advances (e.g., shortened lengths of hospital stays and ambulatory surgery), the dearth of affordable long-term care services, and the increasing life expectancy of their family members

2. The costs of the social production of dependency resulting from national policies that promote neither rehabilitation nor healthy behaviors but that instead foster impoverishment and institutionalization for those who need long-term care

As the new millennium begins, the dominant biomedical paradigm in aging confronts three serious challenges. The *first* results from developments that have extended the quality of the life span without resolving the problems of an increased societal chronic illness burden associated with demographic aging. This problem is reflected in the continuing overemphasis of the medical-industrial complex on the treatment of acute rather than chronic illness. The question is how society will deal with the "longevity revolution" (Roszak, 1998) without either (a) changing the basic premises underlying the hegemony of medicine or (b) creating a loss of faith in biomedicine itself as it fails to extend the quality of the life span and "successful aging" (Rowe & Kahn, 1998). Our society requires much more than fixable genes and high-technology medicine to produce positive mental, physical, and social functioning throughout old age.

The *second* challenge is the inability of the biomedical model to address the root causes strongly implicated in the etiology of ill health (e.g., economic, social, and environmental factors) in old age. The response of medicine, consistent with the political conservatism of the period, has been twofold:

1. To focus attention on individual health behaviors and lifestyles, making the individual responsible for his or her illness (Wallace, 2000) and for "unsuccessful" and "usual" aging (Rowe & Kahn, 1998; also see Chapter 9 on productive aging), thereby shifting the responsibility (and blame) for the shortcomings of medicine and medical failures to those who are ill or suffer from them, such as the elderly

2. The assertion that genetics and biotechnology are the solution to both the health problems of the elderly (including chronic illness) and the problems of the U.S. economy in an aging society (Pardes et al., 1999)

The *third* challenge concerns the tenacious commitment of American medicine and the media to the highly debatable notion that medicine is the source of nearly all major health improvements in the past century—despite the well-documented fact that public health improvements in the environment, sanitation, water, and nutrition are major causes of such improvements. A less popular and competing view is that medical care and medical procedures themselves are costly, are often ineffective or unnecessary, and are not the primary reasons for most of the health improvements and mortality gains (McKeown, 1997; McKinlay, McKinlay, & Beaglehole, 1989). There is substantial evidence that socioeconomic inequality, per se, is a major contributor to persistent health problems in American society (Robert & House, 2000).

Conclusion

The current field of health (medical) services research applies cost-effectiveness and outcomes measurement techniques based on biomedical and econometric definitions, assumptions, and research questions. By not questioning or examining the validity of the currently popular neoliberal theories of the market, individual preferences, and consumer "choices," these approaches serve the economic interests of big capital by preserving and expanding the costly and highly profitable medical-industrial complex. By not posing and examining an opposing concept of the right to health care, the status quo remains securely in place.

In contrast, a critical sociological perspective on social policy and aging embraces both a life course perspective and a political economy perspective that accords conceptual attention to "interlocking oppressions throughout life" (Collins, 1991; Dressel, Minkler, & Yen, 1999; Harrington Meyer, 1996; Pescosolido & Kronenfeld, 1995) as they affect the life chances of women, gays and lesbians, and elders of color. This type of analysis of social policy and aging can provide the insights necessary for a positive response to the three challenges to biomedicine noted above.

The way that the biomedical paradigm is being used in combination with the commodification of aging and the privatization and rationalization of medical care displays inherent contradictions that will eventually bring the issue of its universal applicability into question. A crisis in the legitimacy of biomedicine could reverberate into a broader legitimacy crisis for the state, if the state comes under criticism for putting most of its resources into profit-making treatments of individuals rather than into creating social and economic conditions under which people can be healthy. A critical sociological perspective on social policy and aging can provide an alternative paradigm that locates some of the key factors of "healthy aging" in the society and economy and that prioritizes the production of health care as a social good for all rather than as an economic good that is inequitably distributed.

4 The Transformation of the Nonprofit Sector: Systemic Crisis and the Political Economy of Aging Services

Carroll L. Estes
Robert R. Alford
Anne Hays Egan

Building on the understanding of the privatization and rational-ization of health care and the biomedicalization of aging, this chapter explores some of the major effects of these larger system processes as they affect the nonprofit sector (NPS). Multiple historical events and changing social policies have reshaped the NPS in ways that have altered the "traditional" nonprofit provision of health and human services. Because nonprofit health and human services compose such a significant portion of the sector—about three quarters of all sector expenditures—the crisis tendencies surrounding these services may shed light on larger issues that affect the NPS as a whole as well as on services for the elderly. The chapter begins with a description of a series

AUTHORS' NOTE: Some material in this chapter is adapted from "Systemic Crisis and the Nonprofit Sector: Toward a Political Economy of the Nonprofit Health and Social Services," by C. L. Estes and R. R. Alford, *Theory and Society*, Vol. 19, No. 2 (1990), pp. 173-198. Support for research in this chapter has been provided by the Aspen Institute Nonprofit Sector Research Fund, the Agency for Health Care Policy and Research (AHCPR), the Pew Charitable Trusts, the Robert Wood Johnson Foundation, the Frost Foundation, the Meyer Charitable Trusts, and the San Francisco Foundation.

of eight shocks to the sector, discusses the crises confronting the state, and analyzes the respective responses.

Shocks to the Nonprofit Sector: Historical Transformation, 1980 to the Present

Between 1980 and the present, multiple shocks have resulted in a transformation of the NPS. In combination, the events signal a profound change in the culture, structure, and functioning of the NPS.

The first major shock to the NPS was initiated with President Reagan's radical and successful initiative in his first year in office to cut the federal budget in a new and dramatic way through the omnibus budget reconciliation process. As described by Reagan's director of the Office of Management and Budget, David Stockman, a major goal was to challenge the principle that Americans have a "right" to any kind of social program. This intention was carried out through the first major cuts in federal funding for many domestic social services that, from the mid-1960s to the 1980s, represented the traditional NPS base in the community. This was accomplished through a new budgeting process, the passage of the Omnibus Budget Reconciliation Act (OBRA) of 1981. Abramson and Salamon (1986) and Estes and her associates (Estes & Alford, 1990; Estes & Bergthold, 1989; Estes & Binney, 1993) have documented the effects of these changes, nationally for the NPS and specifically for aging services (Estes, Swan, & associates, 1993).

A second and related shock occurred via President Reagan's policies designed to stimulate privatization and competition and to diminish the size of government. Although the rhetoric of public-private partnerships was used, in fact, policies were instituted to remove the historical advantage that nonprofits had enjoyed regarding government service funding, bidding, and contracting. Under President George Bush, a federal commission on "deregulation," headed by Vice President Dan Quayle, sought a major rollback in government red tape and regulations. Simultaneously and in contradictory fashion, important new regulations were being selectively imposed that, in some cases, prevented states, communities, and institutions from exercising their "discretion" in a manner that was theoretically consistent with the principle of deregulation. Among the new regulatory provisions instituted were prospective hospital payments by diagnosis under Medicare in 1983;

prohibitions against states' having more restrictive environmental protections than the federal government; and regulations requiring, for the first time, that nonprofit social service providers compete with proprietary agencies for federal service dollars and contracts. For services funded under the Older Americans Act, it was the first time that proprietaries were permitted to contract for services and the first time that nonprofits were uniformly required to compete on bids for contracts with for-profits.

Requirements to bid for service contracts at the lowest cost per unit of service impaired the ability of nonprofits to continue to provide either charitable services (free or at reduced cost) or comprehensive services for which there was no specific reimbursement source (unless clients had the ability to pay privately). The successful bidding practices of proprietaries quickly led all agencies, including nonprofits, to engage in service "unbundling"—that is, the selling of single reimbursable services to lower unit cost. This practice contributed to further fragmentation and loss of the already meager comprehensive service arrangements in the community. Also, competition contributed more broadly to other dramatic changes in the behavior of nonprofit entities (Wood & Estes, 1986, 1988, 1990; Wood, Hughes, & Estes, 1986).

Bidding practices contributed to the further fragmentation of the community service infrastructure as programs and services were subdivided into biddable "chunks" of activities rationed to community members based on the number of services funded and cost to the nonprofit provider. In many cases, nonprofits found themselves unable to provide services for the cost per unit of service allocated through government contract. Many responded by trying to collaborate with other nonprofits to increase the size and scope of services and reduce overhead. However, these collaborative ventures were seldom successful for the long term, thereby resulting in ongoing problems for nonprofits. Others tried to "backfill" the finance gaps created through more aggressive fund-raising. Still others dealt with reimbursement rate deficits by having staff members work longer hours.

Competition contributed heavily to other dramatic changes in the sector and to a new type of NPS "schizophrenia" that was heretofore almost nonexistent. Many health and human service organizations found that, on the one hand, state and local funders were requiring that local community service providers work collaboratively on grant proposals and service delivery strategies. On the other hand, these same funders were encouraging a new level of competition between these community-based nonprofits and for-profit providers of health care, behavioral health care, services to elderly, long-term care, children's services, services to the disabled, education, and job training. Most nonprofits found it difficult to compete with larger institutions that had extensive infrastructure, information systems, and financing capabilities. Only a few states in the United States passed legislation intended to create a more level playing field between the different classes of nonprofit providers.

The third shock to the NPS, also in the 1980s, was an overt attack on the legitimacy of the sector itself. NPS entities were accused of being "unfair competition" to proprietaries. Congressional hearings and a program initiated by the Small Business Administration throughout the states stimulated changes in tax and incorporation laws that were deemed to favor NPS institutions (hence defined as unfavorable to small business) (Estes & Alford, 1990; Estes & Binney, 1993; Estes, Binney, & Bergthold, 1989a). Targets of the attacks included YMCA fitness programs, cultural institutions (e.g., museums and college bookstores) that run "profitable" gift shops, and nonprofit medical institutions, especially hospitals as exemplified in the case of *St. Luke vs. Hamot Medical Hospital* in Pennsylvania. Charges were that nonprofits cost taxpayers through their tax exemptions, that they violated market principles, and they did not provide sufficient charity care. The elements of this attack are detailed extensively elsewhere (Estes & Alford, 1990; Estes & Binney, 1993; Estes et al., 1989a). Perhaps paradoxically, even though the nonprofit "voice" has become increasingly important, many nonprofit health and human service institutions report that they are less involved in policy discussions and thus less able to influence local and state policy, even when their for-profit competitors are involved in state-level discussions (Egan & Shaening, 1996).

The fourth shock wave challenging the NPS emerged in the accelerated "rationalization" and commodification of care in the 1990s. The full flowering of the managed care revolution, corporate mergers, incredible wealth creation, and the restructuring of medical care occurred in the wake of the failure of the 1993-1994 health reform initiative under President Bill Clinton. From the mid-1990s onward, market strategies shook the foundations of virtually every aspect of medical care, including the conditions of work and the workplace of all of the health professions. Major nonprofit health entities were converted into large, managed care for-profit corporations, which required the establishment of new health foundations enjoying the assets accumulated prior to these tax status changes. With this hyperrationalization and commodification of health care through ever larger and more concentrated medical corporations, the role and responsibility of the remaining genuinely nonprofit institutions in medicine and health care have emerged as significant issues. A question is whether increasingly beleaguered nonprofit health entities (so often tempted to convert to profit tax status) may be becoming an endangered species. Access to health care for those without health insurance has become ever-more problematic, since the number of Americans who are not insured rose from 37 to 45 million between 1993 and 1998 (Feder, 2000).

The fifth shock contributing to the transformation of the NPS was the overt attempt during the mid-1990s to silence NPS entities through congressional proposals. This included the Istook Amendment Resolution, which would forbid nonprofits that receive any federal funding from conducting activities defined as advocacy (and, some said, even educational activities). Nonprofits that voiced opposition to the Republican Party's Contract for America were threatened with extinction. Severe funding cuts were passed by key congressional committees in an effort to completely abolish programs that funded particular nonprofits (e.g., legal services, elder rights protection through ombudsmen, and those concerned with the aging workforce). Those federally funded programs that were deemed too large, vocal, and unfriendly to conservative causes were in particular jeopardy. This fifth shock is most appropriately described as one of "repression" of the NPS. Intimidating and extremely hostile congressional hearings were held, and threatening political charges leveled. Programs that were the backbone of national associations of the elderly that spoke out against the many drastic cutbacks in Medicare and Medicaid were threatened. The periodic moves of politicians to silence the voice of nonprofits have produced a chilling effect, leaving fear and confusion among many nonprofits concerning what they can and cannot do or say.

The sixth shock wave came in another round of restructuring of the NPS in medical care subsequent to the failure of health reform during President Clinton's first term. It was characterized by rapid and numerous health care "conversions," which created multiple and hybrid forms of organizational auspices and tax status, accompanied by greater confusion about the blurring of boundaries between the for-profit and nonprofit sectors. "Conversions" are a dramatic manifestation of the process of commodification. They threaten a loss to the public of major financial assets of important NPS community medical institutions that have been built up over many decades (Cryan & Gardner, 1999). Between 1980 and 1993, 270 hospitals and 11 health plans shifted *from* nonprofit *to* for-profit tax status. In 1994 alone, 674 nonprofit hospitals were part of various mergers and acquisitions and an additional 140 hospitals joined them between 1994 and 1996. A directly related trend is the establishment of more than 80 "conversion health foundations" that have various obligations to perform charitable activities, with approximately $10 billion in assets and an annual payout of $500 million (Aspen Institute, 1998). These new philanthropic entities largely were a result of conversions of nonprofit hospitals to for-profit health systems (85%), most of which occurred since 1990. Two-thirds of the conversion foundations fund health care, and the remainder fund broad community efforts, including health.

The seventh shock wave is reflected in the rising intensity of labor conflict in the NPS workforce that is partly a result of the lower wage and benefit structures of nonprofits, which some contend border on labor exploitation. This situation is greatly intensified with the growing competition between nonprofit and for-profit entities in the health and human services, which has forced further nonprofit agency belt tightening. Combined with historic norms of altruism and limited compensation, this competition has contributed to a worsening comparative situation for nonprofit workers. The largely female and often voluntary workforce is a vital part of the strength of the NPS. It may also explain the ease with which the sector has largely ignored (indeed, been exempted by law from) meeting various requirements applied to the public and business sectors of the labor force. Labor issues erupted through labor union struggles in the 1990s, diminishing the ability of the NPS to ignore labor issues while simultaneously raising the costs to nonprofits during a period of their own organizational and financial crises.

The eighth wave to shock the NPS and impede its ability to compete in the new marketplace of services is the impact of technology. To successfully compete in today's market, nonprofit agencies must have information systems that provide the agency with a range of data-reporting and data-processing activities. Most agencies now are required to maintain multiple databases of information on clients, activities, services, and outcomes. As government funders grow increasingly concerned about accountability, the agencies they fund are required to produce a plethora of reports, and they often track performance on proprietary data systems developed by the funder. Nonprofits now must enter and analyze data and, in health care, implement complex data use management systems. Other technology standards include the Internet, e-mail, Web pages, and systems for segmenting and tracking donors and finances. As a result, the smaller of the nonprofits find that they are increasingly unable to compete in a data-driven world (Egan, 2000). Technology is another force driving the commodification and rationalization of the NPS, forcing it to emulate the profit sector in many of its practices.

These eight shock waves have dramatically and profoundly transformed the NPS but with largely unknown consequences throughout U.S. communities. From the mid-1960s to the 1980s, a major legitimating rationale for the NPS was that it could contain the size of the state while also dealing with the nation's social ills. With the newly energized market ideology reemerging during the Reagan era (Estes, 1991b), the NPS was, for the first time, redefined as a negative competitive force and perhaps redundant. A number of high-ranking policymakers and business interests made sure that there would no longer be NPS funding "as usual." Indeed, enormous new investment streams funded by the state have been either reduced or redirected from NPS human services and made available to the for-profit sector in competitive bidding wars with nonprofits. Studies in some states show that communities suffer when the community-based nonprofits lose contracts. If states do not have regulations that cap profits and ensure access to quality care, communities report serious problems with services. As much as 45% to 55% of the contract dollar has gone to overhead to the for-profits, thereby diverting even more funds from services for recipients and communities.

A central question concerns the extent to which the NPS can still function as a "buffer" between the market and the state (Estes & Alford, 1990). This question becomes more imperative with the dramatically increased strength of the market-based approaches in contrast to the diminished strength and legitimacy of both the state and the remaining genuinely nonprofit organizations. The upsurge of global capital accumulation and centralization and heretofore unimaginable private profit have profound consequences for the role of the NPS (Alford, 1992; Estes & Alford, 1990).

Crisis Theory

Since the early 1970s, a large and growing literature has examined crisis tendencies in capitalist society, commencing with James O'Connor's (1973) *The Fiscal Crisis of the State* and followed by such diverse perspectives as Jürgen Habermas's (1975) *Legitimation Crisis* and Daniel Bell's (1976) *The Cultural Contradictions of Capitalism.* These and other theorists have identified social crisis tendencies in the realms of economics, politics, culture, and personality.

Economic crisis theories reflect the full intellectual and ideological spectrum, ranging from neoclassical market theories to Marxist, neo-Marxist, and post-Marxist perspectives (O'Connor, 1987). Political crisis theories have been advanced from various theoretical viewpoints, such as the rationality and legitimation crisis tendencies outlined by critical theorists Habermas (1970, 1975) and Offe and Keane (1984). Sociocultural crisis theories have addressed motivational (Habermas, 1975) and personality deficits (O'Connor, 1987). As "turning points" in which preexisting relationships and meanings can no longer be assumed, crises are "moments of truth" that signify "the restructuring of social relationships that occurs when new power centers confront existing structures of domination, the outcome is generally unknown and existing institutions and social practices can no longer be taken for granted" (O'Connor, 1987, pp. 54-55).

Habermas, O'Connor, and Offe have each woven together individual- and system-level crisis theories that integrate aspects of the political, economic, and sociocultural realms. O'Connor (1987), moving beyond the economic determinism of some neo-Marxist theoretical approaches, explicitly argues "that modern economic, social, political and cultural crises interpenetrate one another in ways which transform them into different dimensions of the same historical process . . . [and] the modern crisis becomes one 'general crisis' " (pp. 11, 54). Habermas (1975) has explored crisis tendencies specific to advanced capitalism that may originate in the political and sociocultural as well as the economic system. Offe and Keane (1984) posit the centrality of state political and administrative power for understanding crisis tendencies in light of the state's coordination and "steering" problems. All three theorists concur that crisis tendencies in the state's double role promoting and protecting the market (accumulation), as well as providing the safety net for those left behind by the market (legitimation), are part of the larger phenomenon of contemporary capitalism.

Theorizing the Nonprofit Sector From a Political Economy Framework

None of these theories has dealt explicitly with the NPS despite its size and importance. The total revenue for this sector exceeds $600 billion, of which grants from individuals, foundations, and corporations compose $135 billion, with government grants, contracts, and fees for services making up the remainder (Melendez, 1999). The major distinguishing feature of nonprofit organizations is that they are allowed, under their statutes of incorporation, certain tax and regulatory advantages as long as their revenues or "profits" are not distributed to the owners of the nonprofit entity (Hansmann, 1980; Steinberg, 1988). Because nonprofits have provided the largest array of publicly financed health and human services since the state began significantly underwriting them in the mid-1960s (Salamon, 1987a), they play an important role in the U.S. welfare state.

Although Ostrander and Langton (1987), along with Van Til (1987), also introduce the concept of a political economy of the NPS and Hall (1987) has described crises "of " and "within" the NPS, there has been virtually no attention by crisis theorists to this sector of society, and limited attention by "voluntary action" scholars to theories of the NPS from political economy or critical perspectives (Van Til, 1982, 1987).

The goal here is not to explain or debate the origins of economic, political, or sociocultural crises but to argue that some of the crisis tendencies of capitalism have consequences for the largest component of the NPS, the health and social services. In so doing, this chapter attempts to address both the absence of a political economy perspective in theorizing the NPS (Ostrander, 1987) and the incompleteness of crisis theories that omit consideration of the nonprofit or "third sector." The question is, How are larger economic, sociocultural, and political crisis tendencies being displaced into or processed through the nonprofit health and social services?

Although the formulation presented here differs from that of Hall (1987), Estes and Alford (1990) concur that there is both a crisis *of* the NPS and a crisis *within* the NPS. In Hall's view, the crisis of the sector occurred beginning in the 1980s as a result of Reagan administration policies that dramatically shifted the dialogue concerning the role of the state and the private sector while at the same time reducing federal funding for entities operating in the NPS. Hall identified the crisis within the sector as one of professionalism and management (i.e., the need to rationalize voluntary work and organization) that was exacerbated as nonprofit organizations struggled to survive in a rapidly changing organizational environment.

Estes and Alford (1990) point out that "irrationality" would be expected with the high degree of uncertainty and competitiveness that confronted nonprofits during the Reagan era and beyond. One effect, already occurring, is a degree of "rationalization and professionalization" as nonprofit health and social service organizations have moved toward rules of operation that mimic those of profit-making organizations. This is seen in almost every aspect of operations of non-profit health and human service agencies, including use management and the rationing of care, professional credentialing and licensing requirements, management information systems, business planning, and financing.

Technology is another force driving the commodification and rationalization of the nonprofit sector, forcing nonprofits to invest in technology and emulate the for-profit sector if they are to survive in the increasingly competitive economy.

Yet another likely and perverse outcome is that the environmental uncertainty of the rapidly changing health and social service delivery system may contribute to broader system incoherence, fragmentation, and inefficiencies. The ability to coordinate and deliver cost-effective services is likely to decline. Survival strategies that are "rational" for one organization promote overall fragmentation and incoherence. Market segmentation and patient "creaming" to gain a profitable market niche are necessary under the conditions of pluralistic public and private financing of selected services for specific client care needs. To the extent that such systemic irrationalities and inefficiencies result, new state fiscal or legitimacy problems and crisis tendencies are likely to emerge, even as individual delivery organizations become more efficient and thus "rational."

To the extent that such systemic irrationalities and inefficiencies result, a range of crisis tendencies are likely to emerge (e.g., state policy, fiscal and legitimacy problems, investigations, and lawsuits). This is happening while well-funded parts of the service delivery system become more efficient and rational and the remainder become increasingly untenable organizations as they are rationalized out of the core of the system and to the periphery where they have fewer resources and options.

Health and Human Services

The health and human services jointly make up 74% of total expenditures of organizations classified by the IRS as public charities (1992 data, De Vita, 1997), which represents an increase from the 60% reported in 1984 (Hodgkinson & Weitzman, 1984). Health organizations make up 18% of the NPS, and human services are the largest type, composing 37% (1992 data in De Vita, 1997). Both are important areas of service provision for the elderly.

Changes in the nonprofit health and human services have important implications for other components of the NPS as well as for older persons. Of four areas in which philanthropic activity is concentrated (health care, human services, education, and religion), health care is the largest employer of nonprofit labor (Rudney, 1987). Health also composes the largest component of the NPS as measured by its being half of all nonprofit assets (De Vita, 1997), with total expenditures of $238 billion (Hodgkinson, 1996). In 1984, health constituted 52% of total nonprofit operating expenditures; this figure increased to 63% by 1992 (De Vita, 1997). Education ranked second, with 17%, and human services, third, with 11% of expenditures in 1992 (De Vita, 1997). Almost half (47%) of all paid workers in the whole NPS are employed in health care (Hodgkinson & Weitzman, 1984). Despite the increases of for-profit providers in health care delivery since the late 1970s, nonprofits continue to dominate the largest and most costly component of health care provision in owning 70% of hospital beds (American Hospital Association [AHA], 1996). It is understandable that nonprofit health care institutions occupy center stage in contemporary political and economic conflicts, given that U.S. health spending makes up about 15% of the gross national product (GNP) and approximating $1 trillion, 40% of which is state financed, that medical costs continue to escalate, and that NPS entities receive much of this largesse.

Although much less well financed by the state than health care, nonprofit human services (comprising 11% of total NPS expenditures in 1992) (De Vita, 1997) represent an important area of philanthropic activity because they "constitute the vast majority of social services" delivered in the United States. In general, nonprofit human service entities depend on the state for the majority of their support (Salamon, 1987a).

The authors of this chapter and their colleagues (Estes & Alford, 1990; Estes & Bergthold, 1989; Estes & Binney, 1993; Estes & Wood, 1986) have identified one consequence of crisis tendencies in contemporary U.S. society—the restructuring of NPS health and social services. This restructuring is occurring within the context of state policy changes and economic trends that have encouraged the movement of for-profit culture and practices into service areas that have been relatively well financed by the state but traditionally provided by the NPS, such as home health and acute care services (Estes, Alford, & Binney, 1987; Gronbjerg, 1987). This change is particularly evident in state contracting for behavioral health services for all ages. Many of the traditional community-based centers that provided a range of services have been forced out of the behavioral health "market" with the mental health and substance abuse services either provided by for-profit competitors or managed by them. Nonprofit organizations have been relegated to subcontractor status, providing roughly the same services for fewer dollars. Both material resources and control have shifted rather dramatically out of the NPS and the community as it has transformed them into national and multinational for-profit institutions.

In addition, as nonprofit community health centers (CHCs) and community mental health centers (CMHCs) work to compete in the new restructured health environment, they find themselves in a position in which the market conditions and government contracting requirements force them to create local integrated service networks (ISNs), which allows for either vertical or horizontal integration of a range of health services across different institutions. Successful ISNs develop administrative infrastructures capable of managing highly complex new structures, including information systems capable of a range of sophisticated service analyses required for use management and financial systems capable of handling capitation and risk sharing. National nonprofit organizations such as the Child Welfare League of America and Family Service America and government bureaus such as the Bureau for Primary Health Care have provided information and technical assistance to help nonprofit organizations handle this massive restructuring, once again mimicking the practices of profit-making organizations. However, the majority of community organizations have not been able to meet these standards set by hyperrationalization, with projected negative effects on access to care, quality of care, the scope of services available, and community involvement with other local nonprofits.

Virtually all significant aspects of health and social service delivery have been affected: the nature and scope of services provided, the clientele served, the composition of the labor force, and organizational financing (Estes 1986b; Estes & Alford, 1990; Starr, 1982). More specifically, this restructuring is reflected in the following:

1. Changes in the type of ownership and control of nonprofit service delivery organizations (e.g., from nonprofit to for-profit)
2. Decreases in the number of free-standing institutions and increases in multifacility systems (horizontal integration)
3. Diversification and corporate restructuring
4. Changes in ownership and contracting patterns, with multiple levels of care within single systems (vertical integration)
5. Concentration of the service industry
6. Fragmentation of services
7. Targeting of clients and services toward those who can pay privately and those services that are highly profitable or reimbursable

The so-called NPS has undergone internal transformation that has radically changed its character.

The Nonprofit Sector and Crisis: Hypotheses

Two hypotheses regarding the contemporary crisis of American capitalism and the new NPS are proposed. The first hypothesis is that the NPS health and social services function as a buffer, absorbing crisis tendencies by either cutback or expansion, depending on the sociohistorical situation and specific manifestations of crisis and political struggles. The nonprofit health and social services can "absorb" or buffer crisis tendencies partly because, with the exception of institutional services of hospitals and nursing homes, their funding tends to be "soft," and their staffing is partly voluntary and largely female (Estes et al., 1987). The second, and not inconsistent, hypothesis is that one solution to the crisis tendencies of capitalism is the restructuring of the nonprofit health and social services to expand the for-profit sector financed by the state at the expense of traditional NPS services. If the second process moves much further, the buffering capacity of the NPS will clearly be reduced.

The ideological justification for changes in patterns of state financing by transfer of state support from the nonprofit to the proprietary sector is the contention that for-profit entry will address another facet of the economic crisis—what is described as the deficit crisis of the U.S. state because neoliberal economists argue that for-profits will increase the efficiency of publicly funded services by introducing market competition. Simultaneously, the redistribution of state funding from nonprofit to for-profit entities significantly assists in capital's search for new investments and markets in the health and social services. Some recent targets of proprietary expansion include services that have been directly provided by the state (e.g., mental institutions and prisons) and other services that have been traditionally contracted by the state to nonprofit organizations (e.g., hospital, home health, nutrition, day care, and homemaker services). In health care, the right of nonprofits to continue to receive tax advantages from the state has been challenged by important elements of the business sector. Nonprofit health organizations have been defined as "unfair" to business, and state policies deemed to favor nonprofits have been attacked by some of the larger proprietary corporations, resulting in states opening up their bidding and contracting processes.

In health care, the right of nonprofits to continue to receive tax advantages from the state has been challenged, primarily by the business sector that competes with nonprofits for health care contracts. As a response to pressures and in an effort to create a "more level playing field," a number of states have reviewed their policies and contracting practices so as to not be seen as favoring nonprofit organizations. However, states have been less than effective in defining and analyzing the significant public benefit of community-based nonprofits that continue to provide services at the community level and in knowing whether or not contract funding is seen as covering costs. For-profit health care competitors, on the other hand, are now beginning to drop out of contract renewals when they are unable to sustain an adequate profit. Nonprofits have been weakened whenever for-profits move in to rationalize the system, cream profits, and then leave.

New contradictions have emerged from this absorption of nonprofit services by the for-profit sector. Even though the state's rationale for the initial contracting is to save money, after spending a few years in the rationalized system, states find that their costs have actually increased in some cases and service for cost ratios have declined substantially in almost all cases.

Another contradiction is that successful efforts to absorb nonprofit services by the for-profit sector in the delivery of the most profitable health and human services—with the ostensible goal of reducing costs and saving the state (and taxpayers) money by contracting to proprietary organizations—has led instead to the state's actually bearing increased costs for these services. State costs are rising as a result of the costs of competition (Fuchs, 1988; Robinson & Luft, 1988), privatization and pluralistic financing (Lee & Etheredge, 1989), and the additional costs incurred by the state's necessity to pay for the care of the most difficult (and least profitable) clients. These clients are dumped on the public sector as too costly for either the nonprofits or for-profits to treat or serve. In addition, a number of services are being transferred from the formal nonprofit service sector (e.g., the hospital) to the informal sector (the home and family) (Estes, Swan, & Associates, 1993).

Although U.S. public policies and programs in health and social services have followed the general patterns of development in other Western industrialized countries (Lee, 1984), they have retained a distinctly private character though performing many essentially public functions. The development of health programs in the United States has evolved in three phases:

1. Private dominance, primarily individual contracts between patients and physicians, hospitals and other providers, particularly for charity hospital care, up until the 1890s (Stevens, 1982)
2. Limited public provision of necessary health care services that were not being provided by either voluntary effort or private contract (between the Great Depression and World War II)

3. The substitution of public financing (public provision in the European case) of
   health services for private and voluntary efforts (following World War II)

The role for all levels of government in health care commenced with
federal support for biomedical research, hospital planning, and construction after World War II and culminated with the passage of Medicare
and Medicaid in 1965 (Estes & Mahoney, 1986; Lee, 1984). Despite the
growth of the federal role in funding these programs from the mid-1960s
to the present, health policy has remained consistent with the American practice of appropriating public funds for the support of hospitals
managed by private corporations (Goldwater, 1909, as quoted in
Stevens, 1982).

In the case of social services, voluntary organizations first provided
basic social services. Later, the government followed with some direct
provision, but mainly with financial support for the growing number
of charitable organizations (Kramer, 1987). The substantial federal
subsidy garnered in the 1960s for the health and social services did little
to alter their predominantly private and nonprofit organizational form
and character. Their financing continued to be provided by a pluralistic array of funding sources, including significant private (fees and private insurance) and state funds.

For most of U.S. history, the NPS and the state have been coexisting
and interdependent institutional systems. U.S. exceptionalism in health
and social services has shaped how the state and the NPS are implicated
in the systemic crisis tendencies described here. Attacks on the state
spill over to nonprofit health and social service organizations because
these have long acted as the major service delivery "arm" of the state.
The remainder of this chapter highlights the economic, political, and
sociocultural crisis theories that specify some of the links between
capitalism and NPS health and social services in the United States.

Economic Crisis

Neoliberal Keynesian, conservative, and neo-Marxist scholars alike
have characterized the 1980s and 1990s as a period of economic crisis,
although each theoretical perspective posits a different version of crisis
origins and solutions (Estes & Alford, 1990). Conservative economists
have argued that major economic problems in American industry, including declining profits and problems in international competitiveness,

are due to government interference with natural market mechanisms through regulation and/or welfare state spending. Neo-Marxist theorists have generally argued that capitalism is not only crisis ridden but also crisis dependent—that is, that new sources of profit or accumulation are spurred by crises in profit making (accumulation) (O'Connor, 1987). In this sense, such crises may be partially self-correcting and integral to the operations of a capitalist system.

These opposing perspectives concur, however, that recurring economic crisis tendencies or business cycles promote the restructuring of capital as businesses intensify their efforts to increase their competitiveness and profitability. Inefficient individual business corporations are weeded out, and corporate consolidation concentrates on stronger business enterprises. To boost profits via productivity gains and new markets, business attempts to increase the rate of labor productivity and promotes favorable conditions for increased technological innovation.

The capital restructuring that follows periods of economic strain or crisis has important implications for both the state and the nonprofit health and social services financed by the state. Because of the magnitude of state resources invested, particularly in health services, state funding for these services is understandably a tempting target for reallocation of resources from the nonprofit to the for-profit sector.

U.S. state policy, through the regulation and financing of medical care and social services, has stimulated market investment opportunities by private capital in areas traditionally controlled by nonprofit organizations that promise the greatest likelihood of profit (e.g., hospital and home health services). For example, the passage of Medicare and Medicaid, as well as subsequent changes in the Medicare law, increased governmental subsidies for health insurance and direct payments for care. Both programs increased the volume of services provided by for-profit hospitals and nursing homes relative to nonprofits (Starr, 1982). Initially described as a bonanza that produced a "medical-industrial complex" (Ehrenreich & Ehrenreich, 1971), Medicare has added coverage of dialysis centers (1972), increased residences for the mentally impaired (1974 under Title XX), expanded coverage of home health care (1981), and deregulated home health to allow Medicare payments to proprietaries in states without licensure (1980). These changes have substantially raised the proportion of services provided by proprietary institutions (Bergthold, 1990; Estes & Binney, 1997; Estes, Swan,

Bergthold, & Spohn, 1992; Gray, 1986; Marmor, Schlesinger, & Smithey, 1987; Vladeck, 1980).

The pace of change and the resulting complexity of organizational arrangements in the health and social services dramatically accelerated during the 1980s and 1990s. These were facilitated by a number of health policies designed to promote competition, for-profits, and a health care "market" in which providers have been forced to "compete" for patients based on price and—in conjunction with cost containment efforts—to "compete" on various measures of efficiency. For example, hospitals have been given profit incentives to discharge patients "sicker and quicker" (Estes, Swan, & Associates, 1993) since hospitals now receive a fixed fee for a diagnosis, regardless of the patient's hospital length of stay. And community health and mental health centers are forced to provide a range of services for a flat fee, or capitated payment. The combination of the pressures of cost containment, capitation, efficiency, and competition creates stress fractures for both the NPS and the communities served by them.

The alarming result of U.S. health policy, according to the editor of the *New England Journal of Medicine* (Relman, 1980), has been the emergence of a "new medical-industrial complex" that has converted health care from a service to a big business (see also Chapter 8, "The Medical-Industrial Complex and the Aging Enterprise"). The prestigious Institute of Medicine undertook a study titled "For Profit Enterprise in Health Care" as a result of concerns that health services would "become excessively commercialized, with a growing ownership by stockholders" (Gray, 1986). This pioneer work documented the sweeping changes occurring in the 1980s with the growth of major investor-owned hospital companies and multifacility systems and chains, vertical and horizontal integration, and a breathtaking variety of complicated organizational arrangements, some—for the first time—between nonprofits and for-profits. Recent changes in the structure and composition of home health care agencies exemplify the effects of policies to promote the transfer of state-funded services from the public and the NPS to the for-profit sector. Between 1972 and 1986, for-profit Medicare-certified home health agencies moved from fourth to first place among providers as a result of spectacular growth (4,251%) to claim the dominant share of the home health market (32%), whereas the market share of nonprofit agencies declined (from

30% to 22%) after only moderate growth by comparison (105%) during the same period (Hall & Sangl, 1987).

Habermas (1975) observes that the state plays several roles in relation to the economy. First, state policies create productive opportunities for private capital by securing a system of civil law and regulation protecting the market. Health and social service provision is rendered primarily through policies that promote and finance private rather than through public institutions. Second, the state limits its own activities in health and social services to those that complement the market and encourage the entry of new proprietary forms of organization in the human services. Third, the state engages in "market-replacing" actions as it subsidizes the costs of a private but profitable health care system that ensures continued capital accumulation.

At the same time, the state is decreasing its funding support for social and community care services, although these are the areas with the greatest dependency on government funding (Salamon, 1987b). More specifically, nonprofit social services absorbed the largest losses of state support of nonprofit organizations during the fiscal year period of 1982 to 1986—a loss of about $2.4 billion per year (or a decline of 40%) compared with 1980 levels (Abramson & Salmon, 1986). Overall, between 1982 and 1994, federal funding for the NPS declined $38 billion (excluding Medicare and Medicare, where funding for nonprofits has been rising as the rate of medical care expenditures continues to increase above the rate of inflation).

Research has demonstrated the trend of declining overall government payments to the NPS (Weisbrod, 1998). Government funding is expected to decrease from 37% of total NPS expenditures prior to 1996, to 28% in 2002, and private payments (fees charged by NPS entities) to rise—creating a payer-driven privatized and rationalized system—with fewer governmental supports (Hodgkinson 1996). Analysis of sources of funds for the health subsector (the largest NPS subsector) shows that government funding for health in the NPS will have been reduced from 41% in 1992 to 30% in 2002.

Those state-financed services that are most limited and most severely cut back are the social services—services that are most needed, yet paradoxically, less likely to attract private capital investment. This is because these services are not generally reimbursed from federal payment sources as is the case for medical services under Medicare and

Medicaid. Social services have the additional limitations of being un-proven in terms of their profitability while also being relatively high in labor intensity (and cost) and lacking in routinization or high-tech (generally profitable) applications.

However, even though the funding for social services provided by human service agencies has been reduced, the change in government contracting to capitated systems has resulted in a new kind of cost shifting to nonprofits in which nonprofits are expected to handle a disproportionately high service load with a smaller allocation of funds. Also, the 1990s produced a number of "conversions" from nonprofit to for-profit service organizations as exemplified for at-risk youth in the wake of welfare reform. This was preceded by a tidal wave of conversions in health care as noted earlier as the sixth shock to the NPS (Aspen Institute, 1998; Cryan & Gardner, 1999). In addition, devolution has created new state and national contract possibilities related to welfare reform workforce development programs. Nonprofits that traditionally served those on welfare and those seeking job skills found themselves competing with large, heavily financed for-profits. Some nonprofits, such as Goodwill, created national partnerships with the Lockheed Corporation for training and job assistance required under welfare reform to minimize the potential negative impact of their competition with large for-profit corporations. Other nonprofits directly competed (often unsuccessfully) with Lockheed and others at local and state lev-els. One result is an increasingly fragmented service delivery system, with few cities able to require and implement some of the policies and practices identified as critical to success (Friedlander & Burtless, 1995; Gueron, Pauley, & Lougy, 1991; Hamilton & Brock, 1994).

Each of these state actions has affected the terrain of nonprofit health and social service provision. Reductions in corporate taxation and increasingly favorable public federal funding shifted to for-profit corporate providers have been combined with the increasing concen-tration of corporate conglomerates in for-profit medical care. These trends are likely to exacerbate the fiscal problems of the state despite the assertion of policymakers that a principal goal of such policies is a reduction or cut in state costs due to the "efficiencies of the market." To the contrary, there is substantial evidence that cost containment policies and medical care competition have failed to contain medical care cost increases, which consistently rose at two to five times the inflation rate throughout the 1980s (Fuchs, 1988). More recently, the promotion of for-profit HMO coverage of Medicare patients (Medicare + Choice in the 1997 Balanced Budget Act) has failed to produce predicted cost savings while also launching subsequent and serious health insurance plan withdrawals from Medicare and a national backlash of patient distrust and dissatisfaction.

Other pressures on the state to reduce support for nonprofit services may be understood in the context of the crucial distinction between commodified and de-commodified activities. Commodified activities are characterized by market relations and criteria, de-commodified activities are not. Insofar as state welfare expenditures have supported NPS organizations, Offe (1973) argues that there is a growing labor force, "exempted from market forces," that is, composed of workers who identify with the substance and social conditions of their work rather than being motivated and regulated by profit. According to Offe, the proliferation of such "unproductive" workers represents an "alien" and "nonintegratable" element in capitalist society that erodes the legitimacy and dominance of "equivalent exchange" (Offe, 1973). The growth of the NPS represented the growth of nonmarket organizations— that is, organizations whose raison d'être and survival are not predicated on exchange or market principles of profit and the production of surplus value. Offe argues that "the continuous growth of decommodified organizations . . . tends to weaken and paralyze market rationality" (Offe & Keane, 1984, pp. 264-265). Habermas (1975) similarly argues that the "primary contradiction" of the welfare state is that it is, at one and the same time, compelled to perform two incompatible functions: commodification and de-commodification.

NPS activities are de-commodified labor in the sense that they do not directly create surplus value. However, recent empirical research has shown that nonprofit organizations are increasingly engaged in income-generating or market-driven activities and are being subjected to market discipline through competition (Young, 1988). A number of contradictions have emerged from this institutional transformation. For example, state investment in de-commodified organizations creates the problem that the costs involved in supporting such organizations create bottlenecks in the accumulation process by draining off investment capital into taxes (Offe, 1973). Furthermore, such de-commodified programs create political claims from advocates in the public and nonprofits leading to further demands that infringe on the potential for private profit. Also, as demands increase for more government support of these activities, increased taxes are required (which drains profits) to support the services (Offe, 1973).

A key question is, Under what conditions does the NPS operate as an "incompatible sector" (Offe, 1973) for the accumulation of profits? The NPS provides services that capital needs but cannot or does not want to provide because they are unprofitable. The NPS thus resides in a *contradictory structural location* (an adaptation of Wright's, 1989, concept), which means that in some historical moments it contradicts, but in other situations it supports, capital accumulation.

For example, the growing concern of employers about escalating employee benefit health costs was translated into (a) efforts to contain (by private and public policy) the high costs of health care, particularly hospital care—care that has been traditionally provided by nonprofits—and (b) serious concerns about the competitiveness of U.S. business. It was argued that the price of American goods has been elevated to non-competitive levels by the escalating employee health care costs required for American business.

The situation is complex because other segments of capital—notably those representing the medical-industrial complex—seek expansion of their health care market share, thus necessitating increases in health care allocations from the state. These conflicts between different components of the private sector (between and within both the nonprofit and for-profit sectors) highlight some of the contradictions between the two major functions of the state: the support of accumulation of private profits and the legitimation of the social system of American capitalism (O'Connor, 1973). Also highlighted are tensions between the different demands from different segments of corporate capital, which alternatively benefit or suffer from the growth of a highly profitable but largely private medical-industrial complex and the costs generated by it. The costs of legitimating the capitalist system through the provision of a social safety net (including nonprofit services through a publicly financed but privately delivered Medicare system for the elderly) have taxed business, which in turn reduces available investment capital and ultimately limits capital accumulation.

An important question is whether the contemporary conservative demand on the state to redirect its resources from nonprofit to proprietary services is simply a response to economic crisis tendencies or whether it is also in response to the crises of administration, legitimation, or rationality described by Habermas and others (Habermas, 1975; O'Connor, 1973; Offe, 1976; Offe & Keane, 1984; Ronge, 1974). Because these crises are interrelated (although each may have its own trajectory), the state must respond in some measure to the appearance of each. The hypothesis presented here is that NPS health and social services provide both an institutional buffer and a battleground in both the definition and temporary resolution of the different crisis tendencies emerging in the present sociohistorical moment.

Contemporary crisis tendencies are not only economic. Human consciousness, collective will, and belief systems may, themselves, be causes of economic crisis and/or independent forms of crisis. Sociocultural crisis may be created by class struggle or other forms of political struggles, which may, in turn, generate economic crisis. Crises in the sociocultural dimension may revolve around gender, race and ethnicity, religious, or other struggles. Political and legitimacy crises occurring in and around the state are not always caused by economic interests and dislocations, although they are linked to them (Gramsci, Hoare, & Nowell-Smith, 1971; O'Connor, 1984, 1987).

Political Crisis

Habermas (1962, 1970) has argued that, with the growth of large-scale economic organizations and their increasing interdependence on science and technology, there has been a "repoliticization of the economy" as the role of the state has grown. These changes have fundamentally altered the relation between the political and the economic system (Held & Thompson, 1982). Late capitalist society is endangered by multiple crisis tendencies at the system level (economic crisis and rationality crisis) and the identity level (legitimation crisis and motivation crisis). Habermas notes that, although the origins of the crisis still lie in the economic system of capitalism, the Welfare State no longer allows the crisis to explode in an economic form. In short, crisis symptoms "are displaced into . . . the cultural and social order" (Dews & Habermas, 1986, p. 58). Rationality crises occur when the political administrative system (the state) "does not produce the requisite quantity of rational decisions" (Habermas, 1975, p. 49) as a result of the conflicting interests of individual capitalists and/or the production of structures "foreign" to the system. The state finds itself "with mutually contradictory imperatives of expanding the planning capacity of the state with the aim of collective capitalist planning and yet, blocking this expansion which could threaten the continued existence of capitalism" (Habermas, 1975, p. 62).

As economic crisis is "intercepted and transformed into a systematic overloading of the public budget" through tax concessions and state subsidies to corporations and others, "if governmental crisis management fails . . . the penalty for this failure is withdrawal of legitimation" (Habermas, 1975, p. 69) through the basic questioning of the norms underlying administrative action. Habermas concedes that there has yet not been "a real crisis of legitimation: [because] people continue to vote," but there are real "tendencies toward such a crisis" (Dews & Habermas, 1986, p. 66).

Systemic crises thus do not arise exclusively from the sphere of production but also derive from the inability of the political system to prevent or compensate for economic and social crisis tendencies that inhere in the capitalist system. Habermas (1975) cites a resource problem that further exacerbates the dilemma of the state's role. As costs rise, the state must either "immunize" itself from political claims by the "victims of capitalist growth" or cripple the process of growth itself by taxing surplus value to support the state (p. 65).

> As economic and social crises together are displaced into and within state administration, political crisis may be produced, given the need of the state to organize the dysfunctional social consequences of private production, [while] state policy is not supposed to infringe on the primacy of private production. [The contradiction is that] if state policy is to be adequate . . . it is forced to rely on means which either violate the dominant capital relation or undermine the functional requirements—the legitimacy and administrative competence of state regulation itself. (Offe, 1977, p. 62)

Thus, legitimacy issues about state actions are likely to arise concerning state adequacy in performing its "steering" function. On the other hand, political crisis may displace public attention from economic crisis, ultimately contributing to the legitimacy of the economic system. The argument here is intended to avoid an economically deterministic and functionalist analysis by demonstrating the politically contingent relationships of the NPS with capital and the state.

Two contemporary ideological currents reflect elements of the struggles around issues of the legitimacy and rationality of NPS health and social care institutions: (a) the resurgence of market ideology that proclaims that competition and efficiency are the major (or only) criteria justifying state expenditures and (b) the ideologies of individualism, neoconservatism, and self-help that justify reductions in, or even the total elimination of, state expenditures.

The Reagan administration's negative ideological stance toward government reflected difficulties of the U.S. state in securing legitimation for its own activities in the face of neoliberal claims that government is incompetent and/or bankrupting younger generations with too much welfare spending (see Chapter 5). Simultaneously and in contradictory fashion, the state has both lauded nonprofit activities (particularly if voluntary) *and* restricted government financing of nonprofit activity. In addition, the state under Reagan vigorously attacked trade unions and nonprofit organizational voices of dissent. In particular, federal funding cuts and challenges to special tax treatment and other policy preferences for nonprofits appeared to be a significant element of the state's response to its own legitimacy problems under Reagan and subsequently.

The consequence has been the redirection of state financing toward the for-profit sector, particularly in the more profitable medical services, and away from NPS entities. The contraction of federal financing of nonprofits and the transfer of state medical care resources into for-profit enterprises, such as managed care, are aimed at stimulating private investments and profits with the support of state-guaranteed funding. This transfer has the dual advantage of addressing tendencies to falling profits or accumulation crisis while simultaneously reinforcing the legitimacy of state decisions insofar as they signal a recommitment to the market ideology.

In this sense, the state's legitimation problems have been transported *away from* the state and *into* the nonprofit sector—as the NPS now finds itself embattled over federal funding cuts (Abramson & Salamon, 1986; Estes & Alford, 1990), on the one hand, and its own rising legitimacy problems, on the other (Estes, Binney, & Bergthold, 1989b; Weisbrod, 1998). Indicators of legitimacy problems for nonprofits are growing. For example, the Small Business Administration (SBA) has gained considerable attention for its claims that nonprofits are "unfair competition" and should be denied special tax advantages. The 1988 hearings on "nonprofit competition" by the U.S. House Committee on Small Business (Young, 1988) and the resolutions of the 1986 White House Conference on Small Business (WHCoSB) reflect one major dimension of the problem facing nonprofits. The hearing record contains testimony from a wide range of interests concerned about the "market share" that nonprofits are accused of "unfairly" taking away from business. These include the Chamber of Commerce, the National Federation of Independent Business, the National Association of Medical Equipment Suppliers, the International Racquet Sports Association, and the Business Coalition for Fair Competition on one side and Independent Sector, the YMCA, and Goodwill Industries, among others, on the opposing side. Business testimony underscored the WHCoSB's "top priority" resolution that

> at the federal, state and local level, . . . laws, regulations, and policies should . . . prohibit unfair competition in which nonprofit tax-exempt organizations use their tax-exempt status and other advantages in selling products and services also offered by small businesses . . . [and] . . . prohibit direct, government-created competition in which government organizations perform commercial services. (Swain, 1988, p. 95)

The concerns of the SBA, which have resulted in a multistate program to raise consciousness of state legislatures on this issue, appear to have achieved some effect. Not only has the U.S. government (Congress, the White House, the General Accounting Office, the Internal Revenue Service, and the Treasury Department) become engaged, but also state legislatures and courts have become involved. The fairness of laws for nonprofits on the unrelated business income tax (UBIT) has been raised across a broad spectrum—the arts, education, health care, recreation, and handicapped services.

Some of the most potentially consequential actions to date, however, are in health care, where the IRS has reviewed over 3,000 not-for-profit organizations and their unrelated business income tax returns. It was feared that this process would result in hospitals possibly losing up to 50% of their net income due to pending federal and state legislation to limit tax-exempt status (California Association of Hospitals and Health Systems, 1988). Independent Sector, the national organization founded in 1980 to promote understanding of and commitment to "giving, volunteering, and not-for-profit initiative," has developed a special initiative on public policy on charitable activities (Independent Sector, 1988). Over the years, it has compiled a report on state and local legislative, administrative, and judicial proposals that would modify the tax status and/or treatment of nonprofits, including a listing of the 17 states that have considered or enacted legislation similar to Arizona's 1982 statute to prevent state agencies, including colleges and universities, from providing the same services and products as private businesses (Independent Sector, 1988). The Center on Budget and Policy Priorities (CBPP, 1999) has conducted analyses of state policy changes and has supported mobilizing nonprofits through its State Fiscal Analysis Initiative (SFAI).

Other initiatives that reflect legitimacy questions hanging over the NPS are local tax attempts (some successfully implemented) to remove charitable status and property tax exemptions from nonprofits (e.g., in California and 11 other states), the imposition of city fees on nonprofits for municipal services they use (e.g., police, fire protection, and snow removal), and various challenges to sales tax exemptions. A consistent rationale given for these actions is that the state's preferential treatment of nonprofits unjustifiably gives nonprofits "immunity" from the norms of the market. This market immunity is then used to explain the nonprofits' theoretical inefficiency and cost to the state and to contend that they hurt the economy and small business. Medical care providers have come under particular attack, as the Congressional Ways and Means Oversight Subcommittee has considered changing the tax status of nonprofit hospitals' income from lab testing, pharmaceuticals, and the sale or rental of medical equipment to outpatients— as well as other changes in the UBIT. Also, at least seven states have proposed to tax not-for-profit hospitals in various ways (e.g., loss of property or county tax exemptions) ("Not-for-Profits Prepare to Battle," 1987).

The fortunes and ultimate viability of all institutions and organizations are contingent, to a major degree, on their legitimacy. Offe (1977) has identified three precarious conditions under which the state legitimates its activities:

1. Enough social surplus (surplus value available in taxes) for the state to produce the infrastructure
2. Administrative rationality in providing the right quantity and quality of infrastructure

3. The availability of legitimating beliefs that provide consent to the state and avoid overload of the system

One of the main features of modern capitalist societies is that there are multiple sources of legitimacy for each of the major sectors—state, capital, and nonprofit—depending on the political and economic conditions in the sociohistorical moment. In some moments and conditions, public activity is legitimated (e.g., police and national security), and private profit-making or nonprofit activities are deemed inappropriate; although in others, private for-profit or nonprofit activity is preferred. For example, to the extent that the NPS represents pluralism and participatory action, it has been a source of legitimation for the NPS, just as electoral participation legitimates the state. The state legitimates capital by providing a seemingly neutral and publicly accountable legal and rational framework for orderly economic growth (Alford & Friedland, 1985).

With regard to legitimacy, the terrain shifted in the 1980s for the NPS in the United States, particularly for nonprofit health and social services. The status of the heretofore taken-for-granted nonprofit professional services changed from that of the dominant structural interest to that of a competing interest (Alford, 1975) with state-financed services at stake.

A broad examination of the aforementioned conditions of legitimacy, in reference to NPS health and social service organizations, is illuminating. For example, small nonprofit service agencies cannot easily demonstrate "administrative rationality," "efficiency," or network capacity, given their limited information and data systems, unstable funding sources, low-wage salary structures, and a dependence on volunteer and underpaid labor. Additional legitimacy problems are likely to arise as nonprofit organizations are increasingly pressured to become more and more efficient and competitive, adopting increasingly similar behavior patterns as organizations in the for-profit sector (DiMaggio & Powell, 1983).

The contradiction is that, in attempting to offset challenges to their legitimacy by adopting efficiency goals and acting more businesslike, nonprofits simultaneously contribute to their own delegitimation as a unique sector deserving of the special privileges associated with giving, volunteering, and not-for-profit initiative. Furthermore, when larger NPS entities adopt business practices to garner funds in the more competitive environment, they exert a Darwinian influence on the rest of the sector—marginalizing and starving smaller nonprofits at "the bottom of the food chain." The NPS, although a "complex and shadowy entity" (Estes et al., 1987) historically enjoyed special legitimacy via its claims to represent pluralistic, participatory, altruistic, and non-economic motivations and goals in U.S. society. Major issues concern the continued availability of legitimating beliefs supporting the NPS role and activity and the pressures being exerted on these beliefs under the current organizational restructuring and crisis for nonprofits in the health and human services. In an important sense, the seeming requisite legitimation of the state and capitalist system is a "phantom" phenomenon, because many potential sources of challenges and opposition, such as the trade unions, have already been weakened.

Sociocultural Crisis

Theories of crisis in the social and cultural realm span the theoretical spectrum, although much of the literature shares a perspective that these crises are associated with capitalism (Bell, 1976; Habermas, 1975; Lasch, 1978; O'Connor, 1987). The extent and breadth of some of this work reflects the contribution of critical theory, exemplified in O'Connor's observation that economic crisis "can no longer be regarded as an autonomous process" (O'Connor, 1987, p. 270). Instead, these theories, particularly the work of Habermas, Offe, and O'Connor, demand an appreciation that economic crisis, consciousness, and social action are each mediated by social, political, and cultural meanings (Habermas, 1975; O'Connor, 1984; Offe & Keane, 1984). One of the most relevant arguments for understanding the difficulties facing the NPS is Habermas's view that crises in motivation and meaning are incipient when the economic, political, or administrative systems in the society fail to produce adequate ideological resources required for the occupations, education, and political and administrative actions necessary to support the accumulation process. Habermas (1975) argues that traditional and religious values are undermined and "motivation deficits" occur, as the "reach" of the state's political-administrative system is extended to more and more problems of capitalist society that can no longer be solved by the market. A crisis of meaning is generated because symbols are not as effective as they once were in generating loyalty to the society.

Two types of problems arise. On the one hand, crisis tendencies for capital inhere in what may be increasing difficulties in securing performance based on economic motivations, as de-commodified state and welfare activities contribute to the erosion of the work ethic. On the other hand, crisis tendencies for the NPS also stem from the sources of its legitimation in the human quality of noneconomic motivations. As family, religious, and traditional values are undermined by an increasingly commodified life and an expanding state attempting to stem various crises at different levels of the system, it may become more difficult to secure the performance of noneconomic work (e.g., charitable behavior) by members of society. This is yet another type of motivational deficit. Furthermore, as the state grows, not only may the motivations of individuals that represent core values underlying volunteering and private giving (i.e., nonprofit initiative) be diminished but so also may the legitimacy for not-for-profit initiatives—resulting in deficits in both legitimation of and motivations to reproduce the NPS. The withdrawal of such volunteer unpaid labor (e.g., the 80% of long-term care provided the elderly by family—mostly female—caregivers; see Chapter 6) would dramatically increase the pressures on (and drain of) state resources, as well as capital, forcing the state to pay for or provide services that are now essentially "free" to the state (Salamon, 1987a, 1987b).

The Reagan administration's rhetorical efforts to prop up (and reinvent) the now mythical traditional nuclear "autonomous" family is one response to the threatened loss of unpaid caregiving work provided by millions of American females, most of whom who are, of necessity, in the paid labor market. The research sponsored by Independent Sector, the national advocacy organization for nonprofit activities, provides additional evidence of the potentially diminishing motivations for private altruism:

1. Volunteering as a percentage of the population, 18 to 24 years of age, is declining (−12% between 1980 and 1985 alone), as is volunteering among single Americans (−19%) (Independent Sector, 1995).

2. As federal activity in support of nonprofits has declined (Abramson & Salamon, 1986), the percentage of total giving by corporate philanthropy also has declined slightly (from 4.9% in 1980 to 4.6% in 1988) (American Association of Fund-Raising Counsel, 1989) and has become more specifically targeted to corporate interests.

3. The decline in federal support of nonprofit activities has required an estimated manyfold increase in the rate of private giving to replace the vanished government funding.
4. Tax cuts for the wealthy and changes in charitable deductions between 1980 and 1987 and others proposed (e.g., the abolition of estate taxes) have reduced or will reduce incentives for private giving.
5. Philanthropic monies as a proportion of total nonprofit revenues have declined steadily between 1949 and the present day.

The combination of a relative decline in private giving and public funding has forced nonprofit entities to increase their dependence on fees and other revenue sources as well as to divert a growing share of their resources, in place of service provision, to try to increase both private contributions and volunteers. This raises yet another internal contradiction because service provision is the major ideological justification for the sector.

Habermas has argued that reactions to crisis take a mediated form, affecting social and cultural integration. The "ideological discharge" of sociocultural crisis tendencies has consisted of attempts, first, to reinforce the work ethic, competitive behavior, and the pursuit of private gain and, second, to revitalize traditional virtues and values (Dews & Habermas, 1986). In other words, crisis tendencies and responses to them tend to have a "disciplinary effect" on members of society, with different implications for the state, capital, and the NPS. The resurgence of neoliberal and neoconservative policies in the 1980s and 1990s may be understood as responses to sociocultural, as well as to economic, crisis tendencies; indeed, Reagan policies were aimed at restoring economic incentives *and* social motivations, and increasing labor productivity while addressing the chaotic conditions of social life" (O'Connor, 1987).

Another contradiction is that the same ideologies of individualism and privatism that have legitimated the NPS "outside" of the state and capital are now being used to justify withdrawal of public support of the health and social services, thereby contributing to their fundamental restructuring. Furthermore, the same ideologies may encourage grassroots action, in turn mobilizing political action to demand more state services (personal communication, DiMaggio, February 20, 1988).

Several important questions cannot be answered in more detail in this chapter. First, will the ideologies of self-help, self-determination, and individual responsibility continue to shield the NPS (and, if so, for how long)? This is significant, especially because they may also undermine the NPS. Second, how will the ideologies of individualism and privatism affect not only the distribution of state-funded health and social services to nonprofits and for-profits but also the allocation of health and social services work performed between the formal and informal (unpaid) sectors? Third, what are the social and economic impacts on society of diminishing NPS health and the social services?

Conclusion

Although scholars have examined "crisis tendencies" in capitalist society, there has been little consideration of the role played by the NPS in relation to capital and the state. This chapter has explored the crisis literature in attempting to understand how NPS health and social services may be employed as both a buffer and a resource for capital and the state in response to crisis tendencies.

Central questions concern the use of state intervention in periods of crisis, the ensuing social struggles, and the consequences of the processes of crisis production and crisis resolution for nonprofit health and social services. This chapter has emphasized the links between crisis tendencies of capitalism and what is transpiring in society with regard to different elements of the NPS. Health and social services, a major component of the NPS and an important resource for the elderly, have been examined in relation to systemic crisis tendencies and the role of the NPS.

Following the conservative ideological attacks on the state and NPS, the attempt by the state to achieve both legitimation and support for private accumulation has been to contract out more and more of its responsibilities to the for-profit sector, particularly in medical care. Given the needs of capital for new investments, markets, and profits, coupled with the fiscal problems of the state, it is not surprising that the state has chosen to promote the transfer of state-financed resources from the most "profitable" segments of the nonprofit health and social service sector to the for-profit sector. This raises the critical issue of how to distinguish those areas of nonprofit service sector responsibility that are profitable from those that are not.

One major criterion for profitability will be determined by the likelihood that the state will ensure *both* the market and the financing for services (e.g., funding medical care for a growing aging population and through state policy such as Medicare) while at the same time demand for services will continue to grow. The commodification of needs that fostered the "aging enterprise" (Estes, 1979) and its costly (and highly profitable) medicalization (Binney, Estes, & Ingman, 1990; Estes & Binney, 1989) is sure to be extended in the pursuit of new avenues of publicly financed private investments and technology for profit.

The functions of the nonprofit health and social services may or may not help to "reproduce" dominant social and economic institutions. Important considerations include the following:

1. How the NPS aids in the accumulation process by removing and treating the resulting "social problems," particularly via service ideologies (focused on individual problems) that are consonant with an ideology of individualism

2. How the NPS legitimates the ongoing system by co-opting the middle class and performing minimal remedial services that keep these populations from organizing to change the system

3. How the NPS contributes to social integration by providing an outlet for volunteer participation and pluralistic expression through hundreds of thousands of small- and large-scale nonprofit organizations and associations (Alford, 1992)

A reasonable question concerns how the United States has been able to "get away with" the cuts in human services and policies that undermine the traditional nonprofit service sector in light of the substantial human costs involved. The answer lies in the successful and substantial weakening of the potential sources of opposition through attacks on trade unions, nonprofit service organizations, and social movement entities from the Left. One casualty of the neoliberal ideology of individualism and the market appears to be that the legitimacy functions of the state (via the provision of social welfare and the safety net), posited by O'Connor (1973) and others, may have become more "phantom" than reality.

The NPS is an intrinsic part of the broader societal and political economy and the crisis tendencies attendant thereto. A larger question concerns the degree of integration of the different aspects of systemic crises in and through different organizational arenas in which NPS health and social services operate. The restructuring of nonprofit health and social services underway illustrates important dimensions of general crisis. Indeed, these NPS services represent an important battleground on which the social struggles presently engulfing the state and its attempts to resolve the problems of both capital accumulation and democratic participation are being fought out (Alford & Friedland, 1985). The existence of the NPS would appear to serve dual ideological functions. First, the defense of the NPS provides an antistatist ideology that may be used to attack the welfare state. Second, ideological attacks on the NPS may be used to rationalize the transfer of large resources from the NPS to capital, especially in the form of profitable federally financed service contracts and payments in the medical care industry. In this sense, the nonprofit health and social services sector is a war zone, with ideological attacks on two fronts. These two fronts signify the contradictory structural location of nonprofit activity in U.S. society.

In conclusion, the crisis tendencies inherent in the relations between capital and the state have been transported into the nonprofit health and social services both subjectively and objectively. The subjective level is in the ideological labeling of health care expenditures and the "excessive" welfare costs of social services as a "crisis," which has supported an attack on nonprofit activity, particularly in the lucrative health care field. The objective level is reflected in cutbacks in state financing of nonprofit services, particularly in the social services and in noninstitutional community child and maternal health services, in the redirection of publicly financed resources to for-profits, and in the restructuring of NPS health and social services. Full understanding of systemic crises can be achieved only by the addition of the NPS to empirical and theoretical work on capital, the state, and democracy.

5 Crisis, the Welfare State, and Aging

*Ideology and Agency in the
Social Security Privatization
Debate*

Carroll L. Estes

As explored in Chapter 4, the theme of crisis is a central motif reso-
nating throughout contemporary U.S. politics and is particularly
important for the issues of aging (Estes, 1991b). To understand the
contemporary welfare state, attention must be given to crisis construction and crisis management by the state, as well as to the actions
and activities of structural interests operating through political, economic, and social institutions concerning the welfare state in general
and old age policy in particular. Crisis tendencies of the state that vitally
affect the old in America are being played out in three major areas: (a) the
de-legitimation of the aging and old age policy, (b) attacks on entitlements such as Social Security and Medicare (e.g., welfare reform), and
(c) the devolution of federal responsibility to the states and individuals.
Major negative consequences for all Americans, including the proposed
means testing for and privatization of Social Security and Medicare as
well as the threatened abolition of virtually all entitlements, hinge on
the most popular and dominant crisis constructions of aging and the
war on entitlements (Estes, 1996).

This chapter focuses on the social construction of crises associated with the elderly and the public policies formed to deal with those crises. The subjective and objective dimensions of crisis formation are described as well as the symbolic and material impact that results. The chapter describes the uses of Social Security crisis constructions and their implications for growing inequities in the population. A political economy analysis is employed to understand the stakes of the state, the public, and corporate capital in the privatization of the nation's major entitlement programs.

Social Security and Medicare *are* "the" U.S. welfare state, according to John Myles (1984), Alan Walker (1999), and others. Hence, the legitimacy problems that attend the state also are likely to attend programs of the state. Often called "the third rail" to denote the political electrocution that, it was said, awaited those who would dare to tamper with Social Security and Medicare, both of these federal programs are now the subject of intense struggles of class, gender, race, and generation involving both the corporate sector and the state. The cultural institutions of the media and religion are also deeply implicated in these struggles. The religious element is present in the increasingly political efforts of the Christian Right to impose its values through the presidency and other political office holders in the quest to restore control over women's bodies and to reimpose women's traditional role in the patriarchal family. The role of the media is discussed in detail later in this chapter.

Creating a Crisis

Objective and Subjective Construction

In the past two decades, Estes has written (Estes, 1979) extensively about subjective/socially constructed and objective dimensions of crisis. All of these aspects of crisis construction and crisis management have been important drivers of aging policy since Ronald Reagan's initial attack on Social Security in 1982 (a watershed in the treatment of this crucial program for the elderly) (Estes, 1983).

At the subjective level, crises are socially constructed as a result of social perception and definition. A crisis may be said to exist if it is perceived to exist; conversely, a crisis does not exist if the situation is not perceived as a crisis or if people do not act as though a crisis exists. This interpretation of a crisis does not deny or ignore the existence of objective phenomena such as demographic aging and economic or other structural conditions that may be said to be empirically real and to affect aging policy, regardless of perception. However, social action is inseparable from the socially constructed ideas that define and interpret these phenomena. These ideas are, in turn, affected by dominant ideologies and ways of conceptually ordering the world that are part of intense political and economic struggle.

Crisis creations are, therefore, highly consequential. They (a) generate a climate of uncertainty that legitimates the rejection of old and familiar assumptions, opening the way for previously unaccepted (radical) options; (b) provide an impetus to "do something" while at the same time preparing the public for the idea that sacrifices have to be made; and (c) generate public anxiety and thus expand authority to public officials to act in extreme ways (Edelman, 1964).

At the objective level, crisis creation is an inherent tendency of the workings of capitalism. Crisis tendencies occur with the slowdown or breakdown in profit-making and the appearance of economic bad times generated by accumulation process and inevitable tendencies therein. In Marxist theory, the "logic of crisis" is found "in crisis-ridden growth and unstable accumulation" (Bottomore, 1983, p. 102). For mainstream or classical economic theory, political business cycles of boom and bust are seen as normal and expected. Crises are potential avenues leading to societal transformation (i.e., "undermining core organizational principles of society" [Bottomore, 1983, p. 102]). This is the case regardless of whether crises are subjectively or objectively generated.

A key concern is how crises affect patterns of social struggles (Bottomore, 1983) and their ultimate consequences. O'Connor (1973), Habermas (1984), and Offe (1973) concur that there has been a transformation in the source (but not the existence) of class and other social struggles. In particular, they argue that struggles between workers and business owners (class struggle) as well as other social struggles have been transported from the workplace into the state. Thus, the tendencies toward economic crisis are no longer regarded as an autonomous process but as inextricably linked with larger political and social processes. O'Connor (1973, 1987), Habermas (1984), and Offe and Keane (1984) contend that economic crisis, consciousness, and social action are each mediated by social, political, and cultural struggles and their corresponding meaning to individuals. In addition, social problems and crises related to home and family are increasingly being adjudicated by and through the state.

Symbolic and Material Impact

The symbolic impact is the labeling or social construction of social problems and the designation of cause and effect. One example of a crisis construction with a negative symbolic and material impact is the portrayal of old people as "greedy geezers" who are stealing our children's future and unfairly enriching themselves on Social Security. Linking the symbol of crisis to the perception of old age as "the problem" (and constructing aging as the cause of crisis) is an important dimension of the entitlement crisis. Such constructions obscure other relevant facts such as the increase in inequality.

The material impact of socially constructed crises is lodged in their disparate societal and human consequences. The disparity or inequality in who is asked to make "sacrifices" when a condition or event is defined as a crisis (Edelman, 1964) occurs as a result of (a) the power struggles around them; (b) the ordering (or potential reordering) of social relations; and (c) the resulting (re)distribution of power, status, and economic resources (Estes, 1979).

Legitimacy Crisis of the State

As described in Chapter 1, the state has three major *functions* (Alford & Friedland, 1985; O'Connor, 1973). The first major function of the state is to ensure the conditions favorable to economic growth and private profit. The ability of the U.S. state to ensure favorable conditions for capital accumulation within its borders is challenged with the globalization of capital. Questions concern the extent and effects of the decline of state power and control in the global community over key policy levers that could ensure continuing U.S. corporate hegemony in the global economy.

The second state function is to ensure continuing social harmony and the undisturbed legitimacy of the existing social order (the status quo). The state does this by alleviating those conditions and problems generated by the free enterprise system (such as social and economic inequality of those people who are left behind or thrown out of the market). The state's efforts to alleviate social problems serve to stem potential social unrest. This is accomplished through the provision of publicly subsidized benefits such as unemployment insurance and Social Security. One problem is that both of these two functions require the expenditure of public resources that must be raised from taxation. Together, the cost of the two functions may "spend" the state into fiscal crisis (O'Connor, 1973) due in part to the paradox that at the times when they are most needed, there is less access to taxation revenue.

The third function of the state is to protect the democratic process (Alford & Friedland, 1985). Myles (1984) points out that there is an inherent tension between the democratic function and the state's function of ensuring conditions favorable to the advancement of capitalism and capital accumulation (Alford & Friedland, 1985). This tension is specifically true for issues surrounding economic security of the aging. Pampel (1998) states that "national differences in pension policy programs (and the welfare state more generally) reflect two basic and fundamentally contradictory principles" (Myles, 1984). One principle is based on

the growth of capitalist economies [and] reflects the logic of the free market [where] pensions represent wages set aside for old age in place of current payment and should reflect wage differences during the work life of pensioners.... The other principle stems from the presence of political democracy in capitalist economies. Democracy emphasizes equality and citizenship rights rather than inequality in wages and salaries.... Democratic pressures for equality ... tend to favor universal programs for pensions and other social needs rather than programs based on economic contributions. (Pampel, 1998, pp. 114-115)

To understand old age policy and the role of the state in the struggles surrounding it, attention must be given to the *legitimacy of the state*. All institutions require basic legitimacy to operate and flourish. The U.S. state is no exception. The legitimacy of a government is defined as "the condition of being in accord with law or principle" (*Oxford English Dictionary* as quoted in Schaar, 1984, pp. 107-108).

According to Seymour Martin Lipset (1960, p. 77), "legitimacy involves the capacity of the system to engender and maintain the belief that the existing political institutions are the most appropriate ones for society" (Schaar, 1984, p. 108). Max Weber defines legitimacy as "the degree to which institutions are valued for themselves and considered right and proper" (Bierstedt, 1964, p. 386, paraphrasing Lipset). Political legitimacy is "the quality of 'oughtness' that is perceived by the public to inhere in a political regime. That government is legitimate which is viewed as morally proper for a society" (Merelman quoted in Schaar, 1984, p. 108).

Legitimacy problems of the state have intensified with the increasingly successful claims of neoliberal politicians and think tanks that government is incompetent and/or inappropriate to deal with most (if not all) problems of the society. In the face of an increasingly successful market ideology are the real and profound problems confronted by the state in its attempt (rather, its inability) to effectively perform its "steering" functions in view of the state's multiple and contradictory demands just described. Habermas (1975) described the results of this predicament in terms of a "rationalization crisis" that contributed to legitimacy problems for the state. A recent illustration of the legitimacy problems of the state is the state's own politically defined deficit crisis, which was successfully employed throughout the 1990s to call the legitimacy of state, particularly federal-level, actions into question.

These steering, rationalization, and legitimacy problems of the U.S. state have justified sustained ideological attacks and rollbacks in welfare state commitments, especially to the elderly. Federal entitlement programs are defined as budgetary problems to be solved by budgetary means only (Quadagno, 1999a) rather than as programs designed to provide economic security and a collective community (pooled social risk). The state's responses to its own self-defined legitimacy crisis tendencies include President Reagan's proclamations of the inefficiency and incompetence of state bureaucrats, the abolition of entitlement to welfare in 1994, and the transfer of increasing government resources to the private for-profit sector and away from the public and nonprofit sector as well as massive deregulation (Estes, 1991b; Estes & Alford, 1990). (See Chapters 4 and 8 for more discussion of this issue.)

The legitimacy problems of the U.S. state have been transported into all aspects of social policy for the aging, especially the bedrock programs of Social Security and Medicare. The state's responses to its legitimacy problems are numerous and the source of conflict among contending parties include (a) imposing the ideology and law of deficit reduction; (b) tax cuts for the wealthy; (c) funding cuts in politically weak programs; (d) policies to stimulate the market; (e) erosion of government entitlements; (f) devolution of federal responsibility; (g) deficit reduction to constrain social spending; and (h) a health policy agenda of market stimulation, privatization, for-profit managed care, and individual responsibility (Estes, 1991b).

Race/Ethnicity, Class, and Gender

The interlocking systems of oppression of race, class, and gender (Collins, 1990, 1991) are key to fully understanding today's struggles surrounding entitlements for the elderly. Social Security, as is much of state social policy, is *racialized* (Quadagno, 1994) and *gendered* (Acker, 1988; MacKinnon, 1989; among others). These characteristics are deeply and inextricably embedded in U.S. old age policy. Jill Quadagno (1994) in *The Color of Welfare* and elsewhere has documented the racialized history of Social Security policy, from initially excluding coverage of domestic workers and farmworkers to the higher benefits for workers in the primary rather than secondary labor market. With the rising age of eligibility for Social Security from 65 to 67, there is the added problem of the disparate likelihood of realizing the benefits, given the variant life expectancies and health and economic inequalities of members of differing ethnic and racial groups.

In addition, although Social Security is often described as "gender neutral," the outcomes of the policy are decidedly *not gender neutral*. Social Security policy is gendered inasmuch as the policy does nothing to compensate for the sex-based differential access to labor force participation, the differential caregiving responsibilities, and the wage gap (see Chapter 6). Research on Social Security shows more favorable treatment of those (largely white) married women in the "traditional" dependent nuclear family nonworking spousal role. Women in nontraditional families (i.e., divorced, never married, separated, and widowed), particularly minority women, are most disadvantaged in terms of the economic outcomes of Social Security policy (Harrington Meyer, 1996).

Ideology

As sets of ideas and beliefs that are promoted to advance the interests of a group's position, ideology is used by all political regimes in their efforts to justify their position and impose their political will on others. The contest for ideological hegemony is about achieving and maintaining power through the means of the production of ideas. The political economy perspective advanced here is consistent with the position that "the value systems, normative orientations, moral codes, and belief systems of a society . . . are in fact in a direct and substantial manner connected to the larger process of class rule and domination" (Knuttila, 1996, p. 164).

The strength and success of the Right's ideological political assault on all government programs and especially entitlements is the most successful and lasting element of the Reagan legacy (Estes, 1991b). The twin ideologies of neoliberalism and neoconservatism have been invaluable in the efforts to radically transform the Social Security and Medicare programs. They have been adopted as acceptable and understandable in light of the "crisis of the state."

Neoliberal ideology argues for a "minimalist state" and is hostile to anything that may impede the "natural superiority" of the market (Levitas, 1986). In the United States today, the sanctity of the market over the state, including the "imperatives of international markets (i.e., globalization), and the inevitable need to align domestic wages and public policies with the terms of those markets" (Piven & Cloward, 1997, p. 34) has become the dominant ideology. This view of "markets over politics" is an ideology that has been successfully employed to achieve larger political and economic goals of welfare reform and now provides the impetus for the attempts to privatize public programs, entitlements, and social insurance.

Neoconservative ideology, which has been an invaluable tool in rekindling a gender war, has laid the affective base for increased pressures for family responsibility. As corporate capital and the state grow, Habermas argues that traditional and religious values are undermined and "motivation deficits" (Habermas, 1975) occur as the reach of the state political administrative system is extended to more and more problems of capitalist society (Estes & Alford, 1990) and of the family. The central importance of the family is accepted, and a "crisis of the family" justifies the adoption of new policies that seek to reinforce traditional family structures and norms. Understood from the feminist critical lens of the sex/gender system, the neoconservative ideological current sees women as the cause of the crisis in the family. The goal therefore is the reinstatement of (patriarchal) male dominance and the traditional subjugation of women.

Changes in the state policies related to old age are directly affected (Kohli, 1988). The targeting of what Estes (1999b) calls "welfare state cleansing" through privatization and welfare reform directly and personally has effects across the life span of women. The dilemma here is that the dominant power group made up of white males does not equally share with women the benefits of the longevity revolution. Thus, policies reflect traditional family structures, male patterns of aging and health, and social positioning privileges of whites and males.

Limiting the alternatives that seem possible is, as Therborn (1978) shows, the most important functions of ideologies. They structure beliefs and limit a vision of possible alternatives to the actions proposed by those who are in the position to manufacture the reigning ideology concerning problems and their solutions. A necessary condition of acquiescence and resignation to policy "choices" that economic and policy elites offer is whether or not alternative regimes or strategies are even conceivable. The most successful ideologies are distinguished by their remarkable capacity to shape public consciousness. Successful neoliberalist ideology thus limits the vision of the "possible" to inherently promarket solutions, and neoconservative ideology limits solutions to those of the traditional family structure. These solutions are solidified when the dominant vision is accompanied by a "profoundly pessimistic view of the possibilities of change" (Therborn, 1980, p. 98). This pessimism is created through the construction of crisis.

Gurr (1970) notes that conflict and social unrest are less likely to occur under conditions of lowered expectations than under conditions of rising expectations. Ideologies of globalization and the threat of economic decline, especially the loss of work, together with the crisis construction of demographic aging in pandemic proportions, jointly provide an amenable political environment for the ascension of other crisis definitions. These additional crises have lowered expectations and created conflict in the reciprocal relations between the generations; generations are therefore in competition with one another for limited resources. The lack of attention and discourse to the positive side of the intergenerational stake in relationships and exchanges across time and generations stimulates one generation to "protect" itself from another. This environment creates opportunities for the introduction of policies that previously would have been considered to be politically infeasible or impossible without the constructed generational conflict. The most important of these new previously unacceptable alternatives is the privatization of Social Security.

The Privatization of Social Security

Further analysis of the current policy discussion regarding privatization of Social Security requires an understanding of how the issue is framed. There are currently two major competing "frames" (Williamson, Watts-Roy, & Kingson, 1999) or ideologies in the Social Security privatization debate: (a) generational accounting or generational equity and (b) generational interdependence.

Framing the Debate

The generational accounting or generational equity frame (Gokhale & Kotlikoff, 1999; Peterson, 1999; Thurow, 1999) prioritizes the independence of the generations; each generation is responsible for itself and should not be asked to support another. The generational accounting frame does not recognize intergenerational exchange or exchanges (both monetary and nonmonetary) occurring outside of the Social Security system. The test of the system's validity is whether an individual who contributes to the system will later receive what he or she has put into the system in absolute dollars. According to this frame, the elderly are getting more than their fair share under the current Social Security.

In contrast, the *generational interdependence frame* (Kingson & Williamson, 1999; Marmor, Cook, & Scher, 1999; Munnell, 1999; Quadagno, 1999b) emphasizes what different generations have to offer one another as opposed to what one generation is consuming at the expense of the other. The generational interdependence frame is built on a compact of mutual responsibility between generations, interdependence between young and old, reciprocity across the life course, and intergenerational solidarity. Hence, at its core, the debate concerns whether one measures "equity" by focusing solely on age-related generational accounting equity or whether the system recognizes and incorporates a broader concept of need that is linked to other competing forms of equity: race, class, and gender.

What is at stake with each of these two frames is a distinctly different set of principles. The generational accounting frame advances individualism, whereas the generational interdependence frame advances the principles of universalism and solidarity. The differences in the policy approach are also highly significant in very practical terms; the generational accounting perspective promotes Social Security as a defined contribution, whereas the generational interdependence frame seeks to maintain it as a defined benefit.

Social Security is currently a defined-benefits plan (these plans can also be employer sponsored). Under a defined-benefits plan, benefits are paid from a common trust and beneficiaries are guaranteed a set of benefits once they qualify. Customarily, the guarantee is based on number of years of service, contributions, or other factors. The risks of meeting the guarantee fall on the Social Security system, the sponsor of the plan. By contrast, under a defined-contribution plan, the individual beneficiary bears the plan's investment risk. IRAs and 401(k) plans are defined-contribution plans. The amount a person has for retirement depends on the performance of his or her individual investment portfolios through the market ups and downs.

The Costs of Privatization

In the Social Security reform options proposed by various parties, there are several varying forms of privatization, full and partial. Tim Smeeding and his colleagues (Smeeding, Estes, & Glasse, 1999) have used a distinction proposed by others (Geanakoplos, Mitchell, & Zeldes, 1999) that recognizes three categorizations for proposals: (a) prefunding, (b) diversification, and (c) privatization. With prefunding, the federal surplus in the Social Security Trust Fund is invested in the stock market. Portfolio diversification occurs with the investment in the market, and the risk is born by the system. With diversification, the trust fund investment is in private stock. Portfolio diversification is with institutional investment, and the risk is born by the system. Finally, under privatization, individual private accounts are invested in the stock market. Portfolio diversification is with individual investment, and the risk is born by the individual. The purest form of Social Security privatization is the radical transformation of the current system by turning it into one of individual retirement accounts. In addition to the transfer of responsibility from the Social Security system to the individual for the retirement income available to beneficiaries, there are substantial new risks: greater insecurity and higher system costs.

The transfer of responsibility from the system to the individual occurs at several levels. Easiest to recognize is the transfer of decision making regarding investment. There is also the individual responsibility for ensuring longevity of the benefit. Currently, benefits are guaranteed under Social Security for one's life span. Moving from a defined benefit to a defined contribution results in the potential to outlive the benefit resources. Finally, political pressures may allow use of the accounts prior to retirement for reasons of catastrophic events such as major illness. Such a move would further reduce the role of the welfare state, thus magnifying the transference of responsibility for personal crisis from the state to the individual. Initially, there is an immediate transfer of risk from the system to the individual where a tradeoff is made between the security of a "defined benefit" and the market potential of a defined contribution. Volatility and uncertainty are defining characteristics of the market, and its performance is not controllable by the individual, although the individual is at risk under the privatized system.

Higher system costs are also an often ignored potential result of privatization. Contrary to the ideology of the market, government costs may actually increase rather than decrease under privatization (Estes, 1991a; Estes & Linkins, 1998; LeGrand, 1987). The new costs associated with the transition to privatization are estimated to be between $8 trillion to $25 trillion (Smeeding et al., 1999). Unfortunately, these increases are not born equally across groups. They are regressive in nature with higher costs being born by the government rather than the market that is the beneficiary of the increased capital from privatization. To accommodate this change, cuts must be made in the base retirement benefits in exchange for the hope of higher return. These expenses will need to be absorbed by the current system, thus resulting in further reduction in base benefits. There are also ongoing new yearly program administration expenses. The current 1% lean Social Security Administration cost would be increased to an estimated 25% administrative overhead expense rate (Smeeding et al., 1999). Each of these changes is certain to be born disproportionately by low-income workers, women, and ethnic minorities. However, the Social Security "crisis" and the ascription to neoliberalist and neoconservative ideologies created an environment whereby these increased costs and potential impacts are seen as acceptable in light of the crisis alternative.

Under privatization, several outstanding issues remain, including unresolved problems for disabled and survivors that make up 38% of all beneficiaries. It does not address the solvency of the trust fund that, ironically, is a major factor in the constructed Social Security "crisis" that makes privatization acceptable. Finally, there is a risk of lost political support from the broad base of Americans who now earn the right to a secure retirement under one program that is guaranteed by the federal government, and the solidarity that accompanies it. Two critics of Social Security privatization provide a critical summary:

> Advocates of privatization have staked out their turf on the technical terrain of "rates of return," alleging (inaccurately . . .) that the stock market offers a better deal. And . . . the greatest of all mystifications is the demographic determinism—that ever-menacing "age wave"that serves as the foundation . . . for the entire structure of attacks on entitlements for the elderly. In an age in which biodeterminism generally has supplanted so much of the search for the social causes of humanity's problems, this . . . ideology has a ready and credulous audience. This mystification has helped to convince prominent liberals to join the ranks of entitlement cutters. (Baker & Weisbrot, 1999, p. 152)

Media, Think Tanks, and the Disparate Influence of Pro-Privatizers

The Role of the Media

The availability of accessible, public, and objectively derived information is crucial in any democracy. There must be the means "in which the collective thinking of society can be carried on and in which state policy can be critically debated by everyone outside the inner circle of party, corporate and state power. It is here that public opinion is formed" (Leys, 1999, p. 314). The commodification of the media in which public air waves and resources are "at the service of capital accumulation and not at the service of democracy" is a matter of no small concern (Leys, 1999, p. 318). Such a commodification means "a restriction of points of view in the mainstream media to those based on market values . . . [and that] even public service broadcasters . . . see themselves as being politically 'impartial' when confining the viewpoints expressed to those that are premised on market values" (Leys, 1999, p. 315).

Political scientist Faye Cook (1998) has developed a framework for understanding the politics of Social Security, which she calls "Theater as Metaphor." In it, she places the media in the center stage of the debates among policy elites. She notes, "At the center of the actors in this drama is the media. . . . The media are the chorus interpreting the events on the stage to the audience. . . . The actors seek approval from the public audience" (p. 4). The policy elites named by Cook are the president, Congress, think tanks, the Social Security Administration, private foundations, the Advisory Council on Social Security, and interest groups. The graphic presentation of Cook's framework makes no mention of business or the corporate sector, although her text notes that among "players at center stage" are "financial institutions and corporations" (Cook, 1998, p. 9). Although it is not clear, it would appear that she places business under the category of interest groups.

Consistent with critical theories that emphasize the power of those who control the *means of mental production or the production of ideas,* the role of the media is substantial in focusing public awareness on issues such as Social Security and Medicare. Corporate advocates of privatization realize the value of using the media to the fullest potential in the dissemination of information, the solidification of crisis, and the indoctrination of ideology (Baker, 1999). One example is the June 1999 proprivatization ad campaign launched in 18 media markets by the Committee for Good Common Sense based on the proposition that people have a right to invest their money as they deem appropriate. This position was promoted as being morally as well as economically correct.

There has been little (if any) scholarly attention to the media or the direct conflict of interest of Wall Street and other big financial interests that advocate for Social Security privatization. Such a policy change could make $9 trillion become available investment capital for Wall Street and its management by associated financial institutions. Research must shed light on the links between the corporate sector (of which the media is a key part) and the culture industry of the media—and the "degrees of separation," if any, between them. The most obvious question raised is the potential conflict of interest and/or independence of the media as a major corporate player. Such concerns are only more realistic and magnified with the mergers, such as the recent merger of Time Warner and America Online.

Additional and very important research is needed on the interlocking structural interests, financing, and operation of these new institutions of ideological production—the current-day American think tank (see the next section for more discussion).

The following data illustrate how *one* construction of reality may become *the* dominant construction of reality and the vital role of the media in the process. Equal access to the public discussion should include balanced coverage (i.e., pros and cons) of a given issue. However, a recent 13-month survey of network news coverage illustrates the one-sidedness of the representation of the debate on the future of Social Security (Henwood, 1999). Only 3 of 132 sources appearing on the nightly news were critical of privatization, based on a Nexis database search of ABC, NBC, and CBS evening news stories between January 1, 1998, and February 1, 1999 (Farrand, 1999). Among news sources there was "strong representation by government officials and advocates of stock-market investment—while senior citizen groups and those with misgivings about privatization were virtually invisible. No representative of organized labor appeared over the entire 13 month period" studied (Farrand, 1999, p. 9).

Despite NBC's own poll data (Farrand, 1999) showing that 41% of the public has qualms about privatization, only 3 of 56 "ordinary people" (19%) on the news during the 13 months expressed any concern about Social Security privatization. Instead, the major theme of the nightly news reporting was the distrust of "government's ability to manage their retirement money." Consistent with the ideology of neoliberalism and reinforcement of the crisis state, government officials and politicians (including the President Clinton and Federal Reserve Chairman Alan Greenspan) interviewed on the news "were uniformly in favor of some type of investment in stocks, differing only on how much Social Security they wanted to invest and on their relative willingness to combine private investment with other measures such as raising the retirement age or trimming cost of living adjustments" (Farrand, 1999, p. 9) and on the role of individual versus institutional investing of these monies in the market. Advocacy groups on the nightly news were dominated by the small proprivatization "Gen-X" organizations that appeared more that twice as often (five to two) as the American Association of Retired Persons (AARP), the nation's largest organization of aging (36 million members), or any other group. All the experts and think tank representatives who commented on privatization took a pro position, with the conservative Cato Institute making the majority (four of seven) of appearances (Farrand, 1999). Thus, excluded from the discussion were issues consistent with the intergenerational frame and other issues of equity (i.e., race, gender, and class). The preference for the younger groups reinforced the acceptance of the generational accounting frame.

Furthermore, Henwood (1999) finds that the news segments contained little information even when they were billed as in-depth or special reports. They were skimpy at best, usually running "under 600 words or about three-quarters of the length of a newspaper column" (p. 12). As to the content of these reports, three significant lapses in coverage occurred: (a) There was little mention of what privatization would do to or with the disability and survivors' beneficiaries, (b) the distribution consequences (particularly the "losers") under privatization were not seriously examined, and (c) there were almost no antiprivatization sources interviewed. Overall, in one entire year of nightly news casting, there was little (if any) attention to the distribution consequences or the winners and losers of privatization. Particularly ignored were those who are most economically vulnerable (women, minorities, low-income workers, divorced and widowed women, and the disabled) and dependent on Social Security for a high proportion of their incomes. Nor was there any media voice for the substantial arguments from a multitude of experts and policymakers who are opposed to privatization.

This oversight (or outright suppression) of an alternative view on privatization is significant given the existence of an antiprivatization constituency: Half of the 12-member Advisory Council on Social Security (1997) that made recommendations to the president and Congress was strongly opposed to privatization. The opposition to privatization came from six members who rejected privatization and who called for a "maintain benefits" plan with modest reforms. The second solution, the "individual account plan" (reducing benefits and introducing individual privatization) was backed by two members, and the third plan calling for complete restructuring and "personal accounts" (private savings accounts) was supported by four members. This result, according to Cook (1998), demonstrates that the new politics of Social Security is a "politics of dissensus." The only agreement by the Advisory Council was the need to eliminate the long-range deficit, but there was no consensus on how to reach the goal. There was disagreement even about whether or not to define Social Security as in crisis—with half of the Council (the "maintain benefits" coalition) asserting that there is no crisis and that the program can be preserved with modest change. In contrast, the pro-privatizers persistently called forth the "crisis" and "bankruptcy" imagery. The media chose to present only the pro-privatization information and ignored the dissensus of opinion among both experts and politicians.

Another study of media reporting by Jacobs and Shapiro (1994) demonstrates significant instances of media distortion.[1] The focus of media coverage of Social Security was on changes affecting people's lives rather than program constancy; reform options to cut benefits disproportionately; program problems rather than strengths and security; battles over benefits, financing, eligibility, and efficiency; and virtually nothing about landmark development of an independent Social Security agency (Jacobs & Shapiro, 1994).

The Role of Think Tanks

Think tanks are a second major and growing influence in the ideological production with regard to social problems in the United States. Many analysts of the Social Security debate (Cook, 1998; Zuckerman, 1999) have observed the link between think tanks and the media. As Jean Stefancic and Richard Delgado show in their 1996 book, *No Mercy: How Conservative Think Tanks and Foundations Changed America's Social Agenda,* there has been an exponential growth in the influence of right-wing think tanks. These conservative institutions are both well funded by corporations and foundations and extremely savvy in the uses of the media (Stefancic & Delgado, 1996).

Two particular think tanks have major Social Security privatization programs: the Cato Institute and the Heritage Foundation (Cook, 1998). The Cato Institute describes itself as "a nonpartisan public policy research foundation" that promotes consideration of "libertarian" principles. Both the Cato Institute and the Heritage Foundation trumpeted the "fact" that Social Security was going broke, a recurring theme picked up by news media despited the lack of adequate supporting evidence (Zuckerman, 1999). Cato devotes substantial resources to its "Project Social Security Privatization" and with great results as this section shows. Recruited to the fight for Social Security privatization by Cato are the National Association of Manufacturers, the Chamber of

Commerce, the Securities Industries Association, the Investment Company Institute, and the American Council of Life Insurance, among others. Although Diana Zuckerman and others also have identified the same two conservative think tanks—Cato and Heritage—as at the forefront of the struggle over Social Security, only Zuckerman draws a direct link between these think tanks and the corporate sector, stating that each is funded "from investment firms with plenty to gain from a privatized system, [and they] have worked hard, and effectively, to undermine the loyalty of the U.S. public and politicians" (Zuckerman, 1999, p. 13).

Public Opinion and Social Security

With such unbalanced television and print media treatment and the growing influence of conservative think tanks promoting proprivatize messages, it is not surprising that public opinion polls show Americans shifting to less confidence in the program (see National Academy of Social Insurance, 1994, table 52-53, prepared by Robert B. Friedland). Between 1975 and 1996, the percentage of Americans confident about the future of Social Security plummeted from 63% to 35% (Jacobs & Shapiro, 1994). What is surprising is the degree to which there is support for the Social Security program across all ages and generations despite the unbalanced media reporting on the issue. Public opinion polls show that for the majority of Americans, Social Security is one of the most popular and successful programs in American history and that Americans of all ages consistently support Social Security and the maintenance of benefits. The National Election Study (NES) (Jacobs & Shapiro, 1994) provides virtually the only consistent longitudinal data on support for the program. As Cook (1998) describes it, 93% of Americans supported either maintaining spending for Social Security or increasing it over the 12-year period of 1984 to 1996 (Cook, 1998, p. 11). What has changed is the public perception about how best to maintain the popular program and which actors (state vs. market) will ensure its survival from this time of crisis (Cook, 1998). Cook also has looked further at the NES for the percentage of Americans in each election year who think spending should be increased, maintained, or decreased—finding that the percentage is declining of those who think spending should be increased—from over 60% in the election years of 1986, 1988, and 1990 to 49% in 1992, 1994, and 1996. Nevertheless, only a tiny proportion of respondents (3% to 6%) want Social Security spending to decrease during any of these periods (Cook, 1998).

Other recent relevant poll results by CNN/*Time* indicate that "passing legislation to strengthen the future of Social Security" is a "high priority" for congressional action (CNN/*Time* Poll, 1998) by 81% of the American public, only slightly below the percentage of people supporting the number one issue of education. In 1998, preserving Social Security and Medicare ranked number one as the issue that "will be most important to you in deciding how to vote in the . . . year's elections for U.S. senator and Congress" (43%) in a bipartisan NBC News/*Wall Street Journal* survey jointly conducted by the Republican and Democratic pollsters Robert Teeter (R) and Peter Hart (D) (NBC News/*Wall Street Journal* Poll, 1998). By December 1999, Social Security had moved to third place (21%) among issues that are most important, behind education (35%) and health care (28%) (NBC News/*Wall Street Journal* Poll, 1999). As a side note, both of the latter issues had reached a "crisis" state, thus raising their places on the agenda for issues requiring radical solutions. In many other recent polls, Social Security has been in the top three or four issues. In the most recent (February 2000) poll, Social Security tied for third with the "budget deficit/national debt" behind education and health care as the "single most important problem for government . . . to address this year," but the percentages were very small for all issues (7% for Social Security, 11% for health care, and 13% for education) (CBS News Poll, 2000). Other examples are the ABC News/*Washington Post* Poll in August-September 1999, in which 82% (the highest percentage of respondents) said Social Security was "one of the single most important or very important issues" for Congress (although this was followed very closely by Medicare with 81% saying it was most or very important) (ABC News/*Washington Post* Poll, 1999). The Pew Research Center for the People and the Press survey found Social Security third only behind crime (which was first) and education (which was second) as a top priority among 19 potential national issues (Pew Research Center, 1999).

Capital and the Attack on Social Security

Social Security is attacked for reducing the public's reliance on the market, for increasing the individual's dependency on government, and for decreasing incentives for personal savings, the reversal of each of which, it is contended, would produce major sources of investment capital for economic growth (Rahn & Simonson, 1980). From the vantage of the corporate sector, current public policy of old age social insurance for retirement presents three major problems: (a) They are only at the limited control of market forces, (b) they contribute to the growth of the federal budget, and (c) they cost corporate capital as well as workers. These issues are compounded and exploited through the current globalization of capital, which creates and reinforces the Social Security crisis.

Limited Control of Market Forces

Because Social Security policy is determined by Congress through a democratic process, it is not subject to market forces in the same way that the wages of workers are. Instead, it is subject to decisions made by policymakers elected through the democratic system. Thus, the control by corporate capital over the total amount of the worker's (deferred) wage for retirement income is limited, as workers are shielded from the "discipline" of the market for the part of their "deferred (retirement) wage" that is their Social Security benefit.

The fact that the retirement wage through Social Security is both administered by the state (Myles, 1991) and financially invested in the state through federal treasury bonds means that private sector corporate actors do not retain control over the distribution of the deferred wage during retirement. As Myles (1991) observes, this is

> an event of enormous significance in the evolution of the distributive practices of [the] nation. . . . [A]n ever-growing and increasingly important portion of the national wage bill is removed from the market and subject to a democratic political process, one in which workers, in their capacity as citizens are able to claim a share of the social product . . . independent of . . . their capacity as wage earners. (pp. 304-305)

This situation has the effect of transforming the retirement wage into "a citizen's wage, [with] an income entitlement partially independent of the commodity value of the worker's labor power" (Myles, 1991, p. 305). This "disconnect" between the market and the retirement wage is problematic for corporate capital in that it is a loss of a key area or control over workers and the social product.

Contribution to the Growth of the Federal Budget

Social Security outlays represent a significant and growing portion of the federal budget. Again, these are outlays and public resources over which corporate capital has little direct control, although the more than trillion-dollar medical-industrial complex benefits from elements of capital, to be sure. This enormous potential source of investment capital for Wall Street includes annual Social Security outlays exceeding $400 billion a year (and a total exceeding $9 trillion). In addition, every year a multibillion dollar surplus in taxes above what is paid out in benefits and other expenditures ($40 billion in 1997 and more than $100 billion in each year since 1998) is being added to what has been accumulated in the Trust Fund over previous years. The total Trust Fund surplus now exceeds $800 billion and is, by law, invested in U.S. Treasury Bonds. In 1997 alone, the fund produced annual interest income of $41 billion. The combined reserves and interest income are expected to reach more than a trillion dollars before the retirement of the baby boomers begins to draw down on the surplus. This is an intentional result of Social Security policy adopted in Social Security amendments of 1983 that were designed to keep the system solvent and prepare for the projected demographic growth ahead.

Costs to Corporate Capital

Social Security taxes cost corporate capital (the employer share of the FICA tax) as well as workers, and these costs are expected to rise modestly over time. The shared payroll taxes between employer and employee are presently 6.2% of wages (to a defined capped income) for each party. Between 1960 and 1996, payroll taxes, as a percentage of federal revenues, more than doubled from 16% to 35%. As other taxes have declined and the "tax" word has nearly disappeared from the list of potential policy options for the U.S. government for any problem, any tax (such as the Social Security FICA tax) that is likely to increase over time (even if gradually) can be perceived as onerous. According to neoliberalism, taxes are the tool of an inefficient and ineffective government. Little discussed are the enormous taxes required to pay for the transition costs of the major privatization proposals—estimated between $8 trillion and $25 trillion dollars (Smeeding et al., 1999). The Social Security privatization transitional costs in taxes will compete with (if not foreclose) other domestic social spending; yet they either are not described at all or are not described as any kind of problem by privatization advocates. This, presumably, is because the transition costs are seen as "worth it" because they are necessary to deliver billions of U.S. Social Security retirement income dollars to Wall Street from the incompetent government to the competent market. With it, both corporate and state liability would be capped to all future American workers, their survivors, and the disabled.

Globalization of Capital

There is a definite link between the globalization of capital and the battle for the soul of Social Security through privatization. The brief respite from Republican rule of the White House during the first 2 years of the Clinton presidency did little to turn away the march on the aged and their entitlements that was initially launched by President Reagan in 1983 with his attacks on Social Security. In 1983, Estes first described "The Social Construction of the Social Security Crisis" (Estes, 1983) published in *Milbank Memorial Fund Quarterly*.

The push for privatization shifted into high gear with the 1995 Republican takeover of both houses of Congress. The ferocity of the attacks on Social Security is no surprise, coming as they do in the hubris of conservative politics and this historical moment in which the bull market is running wild. The mantra of the globalization of capital has been successfully seized as the contemporary version of the ideology of the market. This ideology, or as Piven and Cloward (1997) call it, the "hoax" of globalization, postures the inevitability of the process as it is now unfolding and defines the imperatives of globalization (work flexibilization and deregulation) as crucial to the survival of the U.S. economic and democratic system. Significantly, the economic (capitalism) and democratic systems are now blurred as if they were one single identity instead of two different systems, operating in various degrees of contradiction and coalescence with each another (Myles, 1984; O'Connor, 1973).

Conclusion

The constructions of old age and the linkage of aging to crisis in the United States have promoted both politics and social policies that not only reflect but also reproduce and exacerbate preexisting social class, gender, and racial and ethnic disparities among the old. Nowhere has the confluence of the definitions of crisis, the delegitimation of the elderly, the attack on women, and the promotion of reduced expectations through globalization talk (the ideology of globalization) been so dramatically evidenced as in the struggles over entitlements and social insurance in the United States. A critical question for old age policy, indeed for domestic social policy, is who will pay and who will benefit?

A crucial consideration must be the ways in which state policy is ideologically and practically consistent with, first, furthering the globalization of capital and, second, the state's responding to its own legitimacy problems.

Note

1. The Jacobs and Shapiro (1994) study was of a sample of 4,000 Associated Press (AP) stories (of 18,329) between January 1, 1977, and July 8, 1994, and a second sample of 5,476 (of the total 7,218) stories taken from the media forums of the *New York Times, Los Angeles Times, Washington Post, USA Today, USA Weekend, Time, Fortune,* ABC News, and CNN.

6 Sex and Gender in the Political Economy of Aging

Carroll L. Estes

Based on demographics alone, with older women outliving and outnumbering older men, aging is appropriately defined as a gender issue—and in important respects, a women's issue. Key social policies for the elderly have been defined as women's programs (Butler, 1996). Using the social policy and aging theoretical model, the experiences of gender and old age can be understood as being socially constructed in accord with how aging and old age are treated in society. The political economy of gender and old age draws primarily from feminist and state theories to help develop that understanding. The experience and problems of older women and men are understood as products of dominant conceptions of aging and the aged and the location of men and women in the social structure. Both are significantly shaped by lifelong gender, social class, and racial and ethnic group status (Estes, 1979, 1991a).

The framework applied to this analysis is based on three major underlying assumptions. The first is that the problem of aging must be seen as

AUTHOR'S NOTE: Some material in this chapter is adapted from "From Gender to the Political Economy of Ageing," by C. L. Estes, *European Journal of Social Quality,* Vol. 2, No. 1 (2001, forthcoming). The author would like to acknowledge Martha Michel for assistance with the data incorporated into this chapter.

structurally conditioned rather than as an individual process alone
(Estes, 1979). Considering the problem of aging as an individual experience without examining structural factors obfuscates the influence of
the family, labor market, and public policy in shaping the disadvantaged
status and health of many older women, particularly women of color.
Furthermore, individual-level analysis also does not sufficiently account
for the group and societal influences associated with race, gender, class,
and age (Estes & Binney, 1988). The second premise is that old age and
aging are socially constructed (Estes, 1979); thus, the experience of
older women must be viewed as socially produced within and across
the life course. This perspective suggests that women's socioeconomic
status and health in old age are a product of their life experiences. A
third and critical premise relates to the powerful influences of race,
class, and gender and the roles they play in shaping the daily lives of
women, especially as these roles are associated with work, income, and
health. Addressing the reality of the feminization of poverty as it relates
to old age requires a focus on the complex interrelationships and interlocking oppressions of race, class, gender, and other distinct life experiences that produce the marginalization of older women (Collins, 1991;
Dressel, 1988).

The Political Economy of Gender and Old Age

Building on the theoretical framework introduced in Chapter 1, the
political economy of gender and aging emphasizes the following:

1. The socially and structurally produced nature of aging and the lived experience
   of old age as these are influenced by the interlocking systems of oppression composed of gender, social class, race, ethnicity, and generation

2. Ideology as a central element in the social, economic, and political processing of
   the old and old age in society and its gender implications

3. The social production, social control, and management of gender-based and age-
   based dependency by institutions and organizations, particularly patriarchy and
   the state

4. The role, functions, and actions of the gendered state in the context of global
   capitalism

5. The "aging enterprise" and the medical industrial complex as influences and potential beneficiaries in the definition and "treatment" of gender and aging

6. The nature and consequences of social policy and interventions for older persons according to gender, social class, and racial and ethnic status

7. Critical reflexivity and a feminist epistemology (Collins, 1991; Harding, 1996; Smith, 1990) in the production of gerontological knowledge (Estes, 1979, 1991a; Estes, Binney, & Culbertson, 1992), which also means stepping "outside of patriarchal thought" (Lerner, 1986, p. 228) and "accepting . . . our knowledge as valid . . . [and] developing intellectual courage" (Lerner, 1986, p. 228)

The remainder of this chapter is devoted to the consideration of aging from the feminist perspective, with particular attention to social policy, the state, and older women. This approach is adopted for two reasons. First, women make up the majority of the aging population. O'Rand (O'Rand & the National Academy on Aging, 1994) identifies this as "the feminization of the older population in the U.S." (p. 4) in which over half of those 65 and older and more than two thirds of those 85 and older are women (O'Rand, 1996). Older women make up the large majority of the fastest-growing age group—those 80 years and older—the age group most at risk of low and declining income and health. There are 56 men to every 100 women aged 80 to 84, a disparity that increases dramatically with age. There are 35 males to every 100 females aged 95 and older (1995 data) (Estes et al., 1998).

Second, women are more dependent on the state than men, and this is true across the life course. By the time a woman is the age of 65, she is almost twice as likely as her male counterpart to be poor or near poor (Estes & Michel, 1999). Significant sources of this economic disparity are the differential caregiving responsibilities, labor market patterns, disparities in wages and work-related benefits between men and women, and marital status. Older women are three times more likely to be widowed than older men (Social Security Administration [SSA], 1998a). Simultaneously, divorce rates have jumped more than threefold for midlife women in the United States (from 5.3% to 17.7% between 1970 and 1997 for women aged 45 to 49) (Steuerle, 1999). With the exception of being in an intact marriage, virtually all categories of the broad "nonmarried" marital status significantly increase a woman's probability of experiencing economic hardship in old age (Harrington Meyer, 1996). Future projections are for the continued acceleration of these trends, further reducing the percentage of women who are married in midlife as well as in old age (Estes & Michel, 1999; Steuerle,

1999), which will dramatically increase the poverty rates for older women who are never married (Smeeding, Estes, & Glasse, 1999). The dramatic decline in women's marriage rates is a major contributor to the fact that the hardship of older women is *not* projected to decrease with baby boomers and future generations. Older women's persistent poverty and economic vulnerability will continue, whereas older men's will decline or disappear (Commonwealth Fund, 1988; Smeeding et al., 1999).

The degree of dependency of older women on the state grows with their own aging, widowhood, divorce, and associated declines in economic and health status. All of these factors enhance the vulnerability of millions of women, particularly those of advanced age, to the larger political and economic forces that shape state action as it affects different generations.

The Situation of Older Women

The contention that older women are more dependent on the state than older men is predicated on the following conclusions. First, women's longer survival means that older women depend on state health and retirement benefits of Medicare and Social Security for an average of 15 years compared with 7 years for older men (Butler, 1996). Second, because of their relatively greater disadvantaged economic status, older women (who make up three fourths of all of the poor in old age) are more likely than older men to be recipients of the two federal-state programs for the poor in the United States: Medicaid (health care for the poor) and Supplemental Security Income (cash assistance for the low-income aged, blind, and disabled). Third, older women of color are much more compromised in economic and health status and thus more dependent on state programs than are older white women. Poverty rates for older African American and Hispanic women exceed 28%, compared with approximately 12% for older white women (National Economic Council, 1998; SSA, 1998b). State policy does little to redress the multiple lifetime jeopardies of race and gender. Fourth, older women have more chronic health problems to manage than do older men (Hoffman & Rice, 1996; National Center for Health Statistics, 1995; Rice & Michel, 1998), and they use more health services, making them more dependent on the state programs of Medicare and

Medicaid payments for medical care. Women outnumber men by nearly 50% as Medicare enrollees (Commonwealth Fund, 1987). Fifth, Medicare pays for acute care but not for long-term care, which is the type of care that older women themselves are most likely to provide spouses and others and that older women are more likely to need from the formal sector than are older men, yet they are without resources to pay for it (Estes, Swan, & associates, 1993). State policy is thus biased toward medical care coverage for men's illness patterns—their greater need for acute than for chronic illness care.

The Gendered State

The study of the state is central to the understanding of old age and the life chances of older women because the state has the power to (a) allocate and distribute scarce resources to ensure the survival and growth of the economy, (b) mediate between the different segments and classes of society, and (c) ameliorate social conditions that could threaten the existing order.

Feminist Theories of the State

Feminist scholars recognize gender as a key structuring element in contemporary society. Feminist writing on social policy and the state has been animated by four broad paradigmatic approaches: conservative, liberal, socialist, and radical. The dominant theme of *conservative feminism* is biology, which makes "traditional gender arrangements either inevitable or, at least preferable [and] departures from these arrangements . . . impose high costs of social inefficiency and human unhappiness" (Jaggar & Rothenberg, 1984, p. 83). *Liberal feminism* deals with inequalities associated with unfair sex discrimination and related attitudes, but the state is seen as a neutral and basically democratic institution and welfare as an institution that is internally reformable via political participation (O'Connor, 1993b; Jaggar & Rothenberg, 1984). *Socialist feminists* recognize the inseparability of class and gender oppression (Jaggar & Rothenberg, 1984) in structuring inequality, making both production and reproduction in the private sphere of the family highly relevant. *Radical feminists* posit women's oppression as the fundamental oppression, in which patriarchy is the basis of in-equality (Firestone, 1970, 1979; Jaggar & Rothenberg, 1984).

Joan Acker (1988) points out that theories of the state and class that do not explicitly and adequately address the subordination of women and the "privileging of men" fail as comprehensive frameworks for understanding social phenomena. As originally noted in Chapter 1, Acker contends that class is produced through gendered processes, structured by production and distribution. Distribution, in particular, is vitally affected by (a) the dominance of market relations as the basis of distribution and (b) the indifference of the economic system to the reproduction of the working class and the demands of working-class daily life.

Substantial developments have occurred in the past two decades in feminist theoretical and empirical work relevant to social policy (Abramovitz, 1988; Acker, 1988; Dickinson & Russell, 1986; Gold, Lo, & Wright, 1975; O'Connor, Orloff, & Shaver, 1999; Quadagno, 1994; Redclift & Mingione, 1985; Sassoon, 1987b). Acker asks to what extent the overall institutional structure of the state has "been formed by and through gender." Crucial questions are these: "How are men's interests and masculinity . . . intertwined in the creation and maintenance of particular institutions, and how have the subordination and exclusion of women been built into ordinary institutional functioning?" (Acker, 1992, p. 568).

Using the concept of "gendered institutions," in which "gender is present in the processes, practices, images and ideologies and distribu-tions of power in the various sectors of social life" (Acker, 1992, p. 567), "gender is a dimension of domination and discrimination [that is] neither obviously discrete nor structurally analogous [to social class and race]. Class relations do not function in the same way as gender relations; race relations are still another matter. All of these come together in cross-cutting ways" (p. 566). She observes that both the state and the economy, among other institutions, have been developed and dominated by men; therefore, they have been "symbolically interpreted from the stand-point of men [and] defined by the absence of women" (p. 567).

Quadagno (1994) has faulted class theory for its inattention to the role of state policy in mediating race relations and for its blindness to "a defining feature of social provision: its organization around gender" (p. 14). Connell (1987) observes that the power of the state extends beyond the distribution of resources to the formation and reformation of social patterns. The state does more than regulate institutions and relations such as marriage and motherhood; it manages them. The state actually constitutes "the social categories of the gender order," because "patriarchy is both constructed and contested through the State" (Connell, 1987).

Patriarchy and the Sex/Gender System

Carole Pateman (1989) describes "the patriarchal welfare state" where "since the early 20th century, welfare policies have reached across from public to private, and have helped uphold a patriarchal structure of family life" (p. 183). The appropriateness of the concept of patriarchy for work on the state has been widely debated. One critique is that the concept of patriarchy gives insufficient attention to class. Bonnie Fox (1988) argues that both social structure and "gendered subjectivity/ideology" are more important than patriarchy in "explaining women's oppression" (p. 177). Gayle Rubin (1975) proposes an alternative concept, the "sex/gender system," to denote the "set of arrangements by which society transforms biological sexuality into products of human activity" (p. 159) and in which the evolution of kinship structures and marriage rituals has established "the traffic in women" (p. 175). This "traffic" occurs without granting women access to the networks of power, money, and culture because "kinship and marriage systems are always parts of total social systems and are always tied into economic and political arrangements" (p. 207). These arrangements form the basis of the "political economy of sex" (p. 204).

A central dynamic concerning the gendered state is the examination of the contradictions between the needs of women throughout the life course and the organization of work (particularly capitalist modes of production and social reproduction) and its modes of distribution (Acker, 1988).

Welfare State Regimes

Gosta Esping-Andersen (1990) typologizes different welfare state regimes and their principles of stratification and bases of social rights involving varying arrangements between the state, the market, and the family. Under liberal regimes, as in the United States, state intervention is subordinated to the market, and there is emphasis on means testing of income for access to benefits. Universalism, when applied, has an "equal-opportunity" focus (O'Connor et al., 1999). The literature on the "contradictory character of welfare states" (O'Connor et al., 1999, pp. 2-3) acknowledges both the "woman friendliness" of the state (Hernes, 1987)—opening political participation and improving their situation—and the other less friendly side of the state: Social Security/social provision systems rewarding citizens engaging in the paid labor force more than those in unpaid caregiving, workplace policies ignoring workers' caregiving work, laws impeding reproductive choice, and little protection against violence (O'Connor et al., 1999; Pateman, 1989).

O'Connor et al. (1999) argue that the state has promoted an "agenda for gender equality" and has also served as an instrument "for reshaping family practices relevant for women's emancipation, while families adapt to changes introduced by women's employment" (p. 3). As a result, "economically and socially conservative forces" have greatly concerned themselves with gaining control of government and state policy and have explicitly opposed feminist demands (O'Connor et al., 1999).

O'Connor (1993a) notes that theoretical and analytical treatment of gender and the welfare state changed from the 1970s, when attention was directed to assessing the effects of the welfare state on women, to the 1980s, when the focus was institutional and comparative, with emphasis on social class as a major explanatory factor. The 1990s brought debate on citizenship and critiques of "the gender bias" of the apparently "gender-neutral" conception of the "universal citizen" (Jones, 1990; O'Connor, 1993a; Pateman, 1989; Sassoon, 1991).

The typologies of Esping-Andersen (1990) are subject to this same critique: that the citizenship concept is rendered unproblematically, as if men and women experience the same citizenship status. An alternative "feminist pluralistic notion of citizenship" builds on the "notion of difference that includes gender as well as race, class, ethnicity, nationality, and sexual orientation [with] interest and ideology as dimensions of political mobilization and participation" (Sarvasy & Siim, 1994, p. 253). As Sarvasy and Siim (1994) note, "feminist treatments of republican and maternalist notions of citizenship . . . share a focus on how to connect a politics of diversity and of everyday life to a politics of collective common good" (p. 254).

Social Reproduction

Any comprehensive theory of the state must articulate not only the relations between state and the economy but also those between the state, the economy, and the household (Dickinson & Russell, 1986; O'Connor et al., 1999). A particularly neglected area of work on women and the state concerns the role of social reproduction from the standpoint of the aging woman (Estes & Binney, 1990). Social reproduction is a concept that embraces both the work of producing the members of society as educated, healthy, knowledgeable, and productive human beings and the work of setting up conditions by which such production of individuals and society may continue (recur). Under capitalism, women's role in reproduction is the "complement" or equivalent of man's role in production (Mitchell, 1966).

Feminists critique traditional Marxist views of reproduction, which have "privileged" relations of production that men do through paid work and "ignore . . . much of the process by which people and their labour power are reproduced" (Himmelweit, 1983, p. 419), which is the reproduction work that women do that is seen as informal, unpaid, invisible, and devalued. Reproduction takes place on two levels: "the reproduction of labour power both on a daily and generational sense; and human and biological reproduction" (Himmelweit, 1983, p. 419). This thinking has contributed to the tendency to treat matters of women's and men's relations (division of caregiving and household work) as private and beyond the scope of state intervention (O'Connor et al., 1999).

The focus on reproductive relations has two major features of note to the social policy of gender and aging: First, it places the gendered division of labor and the unpaid informal work of women throughout the life course squarely at the center of analysis, explaining much about the condition and situation of older women in the United States (Estes & Binney, 1990). Second, attention to the concept of social reproduction offers the potential of casting a new and more accurate light on the roles of both women and the elderly (men and women) in and contribution to the daily activity of the productive sphere, because it moves beyond the traditional labor market concept of production with its inherent age and gender bias.

The vital import of social reproduction in old age is illustrated by the significant unpaid caring labor, which, for women, has lifelong cumulative (and negative) consequences (Balbo, 1982; Binney, Estes, & Humphers, 1993; Finch & Groves, 1983). Women provide an estimated 18 years of uncompensated caregiving support for the young and an estimated 19 years for adults and older persons (Porter, 1995). Unpaid long-term care constitutes a substantial part of this work, making up the equivalent of full-time work for more than 40% of caregivers (Estes & Michel, 1999). Caregiving, and the ideology of community care, legitimate minimal state activity in long-term care by defining this type of care as belonging to the private sphere of home and family (Cancian & Oliker, 2000; Estes et al., 1993; Pascall, 1986; Walker, 1984).

Under state policies of devolution (Estes & Linkins, 1997), even more caregiving work is being transferred from the formal (e.g., hospital) to the informal sector as the state continues to be pressured to redirect its resources from meeting human needs to underwriting various aspects of capital accumulation (Binney et al., 1993) and to the interstate competition to attract and maintain capital investment. Burggraf (1997) describes the "feminine economy of caregiving" that operates in U.S. society and recommends a model of investment and incentives that recognizes the enormous value and cost (time, labor, and opportunity costs) of women's unpaid labor in nurturing and protecting society's human capital (Arno, Levine, & Memmott, 1999).

Aging and State Theory

A major goal of the political economy approach to the state and aging is understanding how the state *promotes* and *reproduces* the dominant institutions that render older women vulnerable and dependent throughout their life course (Estes, 1982, 1991a). An important consideration is how state policies that define and commodify the problems of aging (i.e., as individual medical problems requiring medical services sold privately for profit) are ideologically and practically consistent with state roles in the process of capital accumulation and in legitimation of capitalist social relations (Estes, 1979). U.S. state policy supports a gigantic and highly profitable trillion-dollar medical-industrial complex (Estes, Harrington, & Davis, 1992; see also Chapter 8) while the problems of old age are defined at the individual rather than the structural level. Furthermore, the "problem" is constructed in ways that emphasize the need for a medical service industry rather than a right to a living wage or to adequate income or housing.

In social gerontology during the 1990s, increasing attention was given to examining issues of the state and *intergenerational relations.* This occurred almost in direct proportion to the strength of the politically motivated crisis constructions of population aging, the baby boom, and conservative arguments to balance the federal budget. New popularized versions of "crisis" were continually being manufactured by politicians, Wall Street power brokers, and conservative think tanks (Estes, 1996). The power struggles surrounding attempts to privatize entitlements such as Social Security and Medicare signify the challenged and changing role of the state in the context of global capital and the dynamic struggles engendered by it.

Race, the State, and Aging

Patricia Hill Collins's (1991) work on "standpoint" in black feminist theory highlights the interlocking systems of race, class, and gender oppression that operate in and through the state and virtually all other social institutions. She illuminates the struggle of oppressed persons for self-definition involving "tapping sources of everyday, unarticulated consciousness that have traditionally been denigrated in white, male-controlled institutions" (Collins, 1991, p. 26). As applied to gender and aging, Collins's work calls attention to the links between the personal experience of age and aging, from the *subject's standpoint,* to the complex and interrelated dimensions of the structural locations in which the individual older person resides.

Other critiques of feminist work in the United States address the failure of "white-dominated" feminism to recognize the impact of race (O'Connor, 1993a). The critique of white-dominated perspectives has reached gerontology as well (Dressel, 1988; Dressel, Minkler, & Yen, 1999).

For racial and ethnic minorities, economic disadvantage and discrimination create serious jeopardy throughout the life course. The opportunity structures associated with one's racial, ethnic, and gender location in the social structure are profoundly important in shaping one's dependency on the state. Particularly for minorities, their already relatively compromised life chances include lower socioeconomic status and higher rates of morbidity and mortality in old age, as well as environmental conditions independently associated with negative health (Robert, 1999). It is not surprising, then, that among the aging, both older minorities and older women are more dependent on the state than are older whites, particularly older white males, due to the cumulative economic and social disadvantage that occurs earlier and continues over the course of their lives (Henretta & Campbell, 1976; O'Rand, 1996). Studies on gender, racial, and class inequality in old age support the cumulative advantage/disadvantage hypothesis as illustrated in the rising Gini Index of inequality within older age cohorts than younger ones (Crystal & Shea, 1990; Crystal & Waehrer, 1996; Dressel et al., 1999; Ferraro & Farmer, 1996).

Social Class, Gender, and Aging

Consideration needs to be given both to the differential implications of retirement and old age by gender and to the implications of retirement and old age *for* class relationships—and both according to racial and ethnic status. The fact that most of the aged must face life on a fixed income is a reflection of class relations and a factor in the analysis of class and aging, the processes of social control (e.g., welfare and middle-class entitlements such as Medicare), and the social integration of the elderly (e.g., democratic processes).

Questions of age and social class are further illuminated when gender is explicitly taken into account. Are older women in their own or in their husband's social class, and is this the class of pre-retirement "origin" (e.g., in younger age) or the social class of "destination" in old age (e.g., based on retirement income and assets)? When an older male spouse dies, the economic status of the surviving female spouse often changes dramatically, usually negatively (Burkhauser & Smeeding, 1994). Divorce usually precipitates a similar result for women. For an older woman experiencing such changes in marital status (e.g., widowhood or divorce), is her social class derived from (or mediated by) the class of her (former or late) husband or from her own (likely, downwardly mobile) direct relation to productively derived resources? The issue of direct and mediated class location is profoundly important (Wright, 1989, 1997) and has implications both for social class identification and for the "treatment" of the condition of older women through state policy.

The dependent status of many older persons subjects them to a greater degree than younger persons to the social relations of subordination to public and private service agencies that act to reproduce capitalist culture and class relations. Analyses of class and age need to be concerned with understanding how individual elders, given their unique biographies and historical moment, are made differentially dependent according to their pre-retirement social class, gender, racial, and ethnic status. For example, a "differential process of devaluation" occurs based on class and gender (Nelson, 1995). Working-class elders, particularly minority elders, are more rapidly devalued in the labor market and in the society as a whole than are the aged of other classes. Similarly, women, whose daily work and labor are not generally considered productive, and whose physical beauty is defined by youth, are more devalued than men in old age (Estes & Binney, 1990); Cancian and Oliker (2000) and others note the significant devaluation of caring work.

Women's Roles, Social Institutions, and Social Policy

An examination of women's roles in society as caregivers, workers, and citizens and beneficiaries of social policy is central to the study of gender and aging. These roles are neither inclusive nor mutually exclusive; they form a complex and dynamic interrelationship. Women's different roles have corresponding institutional structures that mediate between them as individuals and society (see Table 6.1).

The family, mainly with the support of the unpaid labor of women, continues to be the institution that assumes primary responsibility for the young and the old; however, as noted, the family does not operate in isolation of the labor market and the state. Women are linked to the state in three types of status: as citizens with political rights, as clients and consumers of welfare state services, and as employees in the state sector (Estes, Gerard, Zones, & Swan, 1984; Hernes, 1987; Jones & Estes, 1997; Sassoon, 1987b).

Madonna Harrington Meyer (1990) observes that a "gender sensitive approach" to analysis of the state and old age is attentive to the sources of bias in state policy that are disadvantageous to women. This is contrasted with a class-based focus that attends to how the state affects citizens of different social classes and a race-based focus concerned with the effects of welfare state regimes on racial and ethnic minorities.

Table 6.1. Women's Roles

Women's Roles	Institutional Structure
Caregivers	Family/marriage
Workers	Labor market
Citizens/beneficiaries	The state and social policy

SOURCES: Estes, Gerard, Zones, and Swan (1984) and Jones and Estes (1997).

All three perspectives are essential to understanding the social justice claims and issues that face older women. Harrington Meyer also contributes to a line of U.S. and British feminist writing in suggesting that old-age income schemes are gendered in three key ways: (a) Retirement income is linked to waged labor, which is itself gendered; (b) nonwaged reproductive labor, performed predominantly by women, is not recognized as labor and as a woman's own original contribution; and (c) "family status is conceptualized as permanent rather than transient (when it is neither)" (Harrington Meyer, 1990, p. 551).

Under conservative political regimes, increasing attention is being given to women's family and caregiving responsibilities and their responsibility for procreation. In the U.S. case, this is occurring through the increasingly violent anti-abortion movement, which, at the extreme, defines all forms of birth control as abortions equivalent to murder. With more women working and the demographic boom ahead, the pressures to continue—and even increase—women's reproductive labor via their "free" long-term caregiving for the elderly are a vital concern of women of all ages. Indeed, how much more unpaid caregiving work and responsibility is it reasonable to demand, when families (women) already provide 80% of the care and about 80% of long-term care recipients receive 100% of this care in the informal rather than the formal sector? The value of this caregiving in the United States is substantial, estimated at $196 billion in 1997, calculated at the wage rate of a mere $8.18 per hour (Arno et al., 1999). Based on research, the average caregiver spends 17.9 hours a week on caregiving (Estes & Michel, 1999). For a more extensive examination of health work and caregiving, see Chapter 11.

Pascall (1986) observes that the state sustains the subordination of women through social policy based on a particular family form—the nuclear family with a male breadwinner and a dependent wife. State retirement policy under Social Security that rewards the increasingly rare, but intact, "traditional" nuclear family (Harrington Meyer, 1996) imposes a normative and preferential view of the family that is inherently disadvantageous to the majority of the elderly (older women). This is so because Social Security benefits are higher for married than nonmarried persons and for nonworking dependent spouses than for working nondependent spouses and/or single individuals (who are more likely to be women than men).

Dependent relations are sustained by Social Security and other agencies of the welfare state that lock women into a spousal wage relationship. The state also supports this relationship through the labor market and the refusal to pay for the caring work of women. "The price of such caring work is economic dependence . . . [which] amounts to the exploitation of one kind of dependency to deal with another" (Pascall, 1986, p. 29). Harrington Meyer (1990) further explains:

[The] paradox for women is either to live without a male wage and risk impoverishment or to live with a male wage and risk dependency. Policies that deny the realities of women's lives by assuming or forcing economic independence ignore the economic dependency associated with reproductive labor under the current system. Yet policies that recognize women's economic dependency also sustain that dependency. . . . The gendered structure of waged labor, the gendered definition of work, and the conceptualization of family status as permanent rather than transient all intersect to impoverish old women. (pp. 560-561)

Thus, the gendered status of working and retirement wages has resulted in women's dependency on the "family wage" of a male breadwinner. Although "supposedly designed to provide economic security to dependent wives, [the family wage] has historically served to increase men's status in both the labor market and the family. [Furthermore,] in the eyes of the State, it does not belong to [women] . . . in the case of marital dissolution" (p. 559).

Conclusion

Social policy contributes to the dependency of older women. This dependency is socially produced as a result of four factors. First, women's roles and treatment in the family, market, and state are characterized by (a) gendered policy in the public and private sectors, (b) wage inequality and sex discrimination, and (c) reproductive labor that is not financially remunerated. Second, medical care policy provides public financing for acute care but not for long-term or chronic illness and supportive care that women need. Third, the state refuses both (a) to recognize or compensate for years of reproductive (informal care-giving) labor under Social Security retirement policy and (b) to adopt a universal state policy of long-term care, thus requiring women to do the caregiving work (unpaid). Fourth, social policy reflects the dominant ideologies and belief systems operating under the liberal state policies of the United States that enforce, bolster, and extend the structure of white male advantage and the social disadvantage of women, particularly women of color in the larger economic, political, and social order. This occurs through gendered institutions (Acker 1992).

A critical perspective on gender, social policy, and aging requires both a life course perspective and the political economy perspective (Dressel et al., 1999; Harrington Meyer, 1996; Pescosolido & Kronenfeld, 1995). The life course perspective accords needed conceptual attention to "interlocking oppressions throughout life" (Dressel et al., 1999) as they affect one's and one's group's life chances and as they are processed through gendered institutions, including the state, the economic system, and the sex/gender system. As Pescosolido and Kronenfeld (1995) argue, the life course perspective is an alternative model for understanding access to health care and health insurance, in which the "interplay of paid and unpaid work, labor market and family characteristics and structural and individual determinants of access to health insurance" is considered (Elder, 1992; Hagestad, 1990; Harrington Meyer, 1996). More important, this approach links family and work with health care access across the life course, with both seen as dynamic and cumulative in their effects. This perspective builds on Collins's (1991) observation that gender, race, class, and age represent interlocking systems of inequality—"interrelated axes of social structure" and not just "separate features of experience." The relationships between and among social class, gender, race, ethnicity, and age—and the subjective and objective experiences of them—are significant theoretical and empirical problems to be addressed at all levels of analysis (macro, meso, and micro) in present and future work on the political economy of gender and aging.

7 Inequality and Aging

The Creation of Dependency

Chiquita A. Collins
Carroll L. Estes
Julia E. Bradsher

Creating Dependency

Dependency can be a matter of both *social* definition—of society's or the medical profession's defining and treating an individual as dependent—and *self*-definition—of seeing oneself as helpless, powerless, or needy (Munnichs & van den Heuvel, 1976). Dependency is commonly treated in the literature as a function of individual lifetime choices about education, work skills, occupation, savings, and economic resources (Clark & Spengler, 1980). This says little, however, about the social context of dependency and even less about the social production or construction of dependency. Dependency "always has reference to a social relationship in which it occurs" (Munnichs & van den Heuvel, 1976, p. 165). Although negative connotations of dependency are deeply rooted in the national psyche, the phenomenon of dependency is not necessarily undesirable. Mutual dependence (or interdependence) is necessary to form and maintain human relationships. Munnichs and

AUTHORS' NOTE: The authors acknowledge that this chapter draws on some material from Chapter 5 in *Political Economy, Health, and Aging,* by C. L. Estes, L. Gerard, J. S. Zones, and J. Swan (Boston: Little, Brown, 1984). We thank Jane Sprague Zones for some of the insights included in this chapter. The authors would like to acknowledge Dorothy P. Rice for assistance with the health statistics data incorporated into this chapter.

van den Heuvel (1976), for example, find interdependency more descriptive of "the concrete situation in which many people find themselves than the polar extremes of independence or dependence" (p. 4).

In the 21st century with its demographic changes, the issues of individual and population dependency are paramount. Dependency is not a "given" but is a product of both intrinsic and extrinsic aging; that is, an as yet undetermined (but significant) amount of dependency is modifiable, preventable, or reversible (Rowe & Kahn, 1987, 1998). The problem of dependency among the elderly needs to be understood in terms of its origins. Dependency is an inherently social product (Estes, 1979; Estes & Alford, 1990; Townsend, 1981; Walker, 1980), which can easily be understood in terms of the effects of public policy. For example, without Social Security, older persons as a group would be impoverished and economically dependent—not because of lack of planning but because the economy is organized according to differential rewards for productive labor, from which elders are generally and systematically excluded through retirement (Estes, Gerard, Zones, & Swan, 1984). Similarly, without Medicare, a much larger segment of the older population would be more economically and/or physically dependent because of their full exposure to the unaffordability of medical care.

As a social product, dependency of the elderly is constructed by a multitude of social forces (Estes, 1979, 1993). Dependency may be produced by low self-esteem, loss of a sense of personal control, or lack of self-confidence resulting from the stigmatized status of older persons in our society (Rodin & Langer, 1977). The asymmetrical power relations and social distance between older persons and the professional caregivers who provide services to them may also produce dependency (Estes, 1979; Phillipson & Walker, 1986). Professionals and service providers may function as "moral overseers" (Zola, 1975) who shape and manipulate the behavior of elderly people (and the perceptions and treatment of older persons by others). The power inequities between providers and patients and elder social disenfranchisement may be seen at their worst in the authoritarian regimes that operate in nursing homes, on some hospital wards, in residential care homes, and wherever there is belittling and demeaning behavior of caregivers toward elders.

Walker's (1980) analysis of the social creation of dependency in old age underscores the point that many complex social, political, and economic forces are called into play that may contribute to the production of dependency (rather than its reduction) in old age. Myles concurs, in the sense that

> old age and "old people" as we now know them are an *effect*, not a cause of the welfare state. Withdrawal from the labor force in advance of physiological old age—the institutionalization of retirement and the creation of a new social category of superannuated elders, especially within the working class—occurred after and was made possible by the invention of old age pensions and other welfare state programs. (quoted by Graebner, 1980, p. 7)

Public and private sector policies, social norms, and other social practices contribute to the dependency of older persons, including the following:

1. Social policies and practices that have permitted age discrimination and, until recently, mandatory retirement
2. Public policy that does not provide full income replacement for persons in retirement (hence, generally provides elders with lower retirement incomes than their working wages)
3. The fact that Medicare covers acute medical care but does not cover long-term social and personal support in the home and community needed by the functionally disabled and chronically ill
4. The declining income of persons with increasing age as they spend down assets to pay for their health care costs (e.g., out-of-pocket prescription drug costs) not covered by Medicare
5. The exclusion of elders from multiple arenas of social life accompanying the losses of retirement, widowhood, and the death of one's age peers

Finally, exposure to institutional racism, sexism, and other forms of social disadvantage and their consequences in old age renders older persons of color and women, in particular, vulnerable to economic dependency, which, in turn, limits their options on a number of fronts.

Despite the need for a broad-based social approach, health and social policy interventions have largely focused on those factors that can be altered by the exercise of individual choice. The federal government has set health objectives consistent with this approach in its *Healthy People 2000 National Health Promotion and Disease Prevention Objectives* (Lee, 2000), including (a) increasing the healthy life span for all Americans, (b) reducing health disparities among Americans, and

(c) achieving access to preventive health care services for all Americans. In contrast, the politico-economic context of aging and health, although potentially subject to intervention, is not easily modified by the efforts of the individuals acting separately and in isolation from one another (see Chapter 9 on productive aging).

Population Growth and the Dependency Ratio

The overall picture of American elders is one of rapid growth, which includes large numbers of the oldest old with growing health- and disability-related needs, and major sectors, particularly defined by race and gender, with inadequate resources to meet those needs. The fear that the growing older population will place catastrophic burdens on society and deplete health care resources has been termed "apocalyptic demography" (Robertson, 1990). This fear and the shape of the long-term system designed to meet the needs of elders are deeply affected by the political economy of society.

Demographic Changes

The "graying of America" or the demographic shift in the age composition—from a relatively young (14 years of age or younger) to an elderly population (65 years or over)—of the United States is well documented. The proportion of the population over 65 is projected to more than double in the next 50 years. In 1990, there were 31.1 million people aged 65 and older, and that number is estimated to increase to 82.0 million by 2050 (U.S. Bureau of the Census, 2000). Of equal importance, the U.S. population is becoming increasingly diverse, with racial and ethnic diversity among the elderly growing substantially in the coming decades. In 1990, Hispanic and minority groups—non-Hispanic blacks, Asians/Pacific Islanders, and American Indians—made up 25% of the U.S. population. The U.S. Bureau of the Census projects that these groups will represent almost half of the U.S. population by 2050 if levels of fertility, mortality, and net migration follow recent trends. At the same time that the overall population becomes more diverse, a greater proportion of the elderly will become more racially and ethnically diverse.

As shown in Figure 7.1, in 1995 non-Hispanic whites accounted for 85% of the total elderly population, a proportion expected to substantially decline by 2050. Over this period, the proportion of elderly Hispanics is expected to triple (from 5% to 16%). Blacks would increase from 8% to 10%. Asians/Pacific Islanders, American Indians, Eskimos, and Aleuts combined would increase from 2.4% of the total elderly population to 7.6% over the 1995 to 2050 period. In addition to its rapid growth, the elderly population is itself aging. The "oldest old," or persons aged 85 years and over, make up a small but rapidly growing group. In 1994, 3 million Americans were 85 years or older and represented nearly 10% of the elderly population (U.S. Bureau of the Census, 1996). According to the Census Bureau's "middle series" projections, those aged 85 and over will more than quadruple between 2000 and 2050, to 19 million, constituting 24% of the elderly (U.S. Bureau of the Census, 2000). Also noteworthy are trends in the number of racial and ethnic minority individuals in this age group. The Bureau of the Census projects that by 2050, the number of non-Hispanic blacks aged 85 and older will increase to 1.9 million. It is estimated that Hispanics will number 2.6 million, and other minorities, 1.1 million (U.S. Bureau of the Census, 2000).

The "Impending" Health Care "Crisis"

The graying of America has led some to conclude that health care in the United States is in a state of "crisis" and that the elderly are a major contributing factor (Estes, Swan, & associates, 1993). Both health services costs and use rise with age.

The total national health expenditures were $1.15 trillion and were more than 13.5% of the nation's gross national product (GNP) in 1998 (Health Care Financing Administration [HCFA], 1998a). This is 364.7% higher than costs in 1980 when health care was 8.9% of the GNP. National health care expenditures are projected to double to $2.18 trillion or 16.2% of the GNP by 2008 (HCFA, 1998b). Despite policies designed to promote competition and cost containment, national health expenditures grew at an annual average rate of 11% in the 1980s and at a 5% rate from 1990 to 1997 (the early wave of managed care) (U.S. Department of Health and Human Services [DHHS], 1999). These costs have continued to rise well above the inflation rate and to

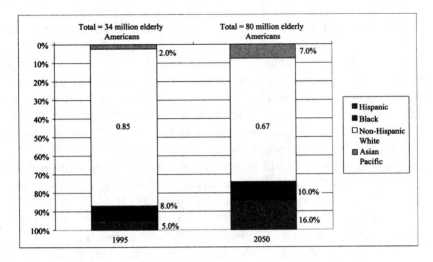

Figure 7.1. Racial and Ethnic Composition of Individuals Aged 65 and Older, 1995 and 2050

SOURCE: Tres (1995).

rise faster than the overall economy. If current trends continue, medical costs could exceed 30% of the nation's GNP by 2020.

Health care costs are not just societal; they also affect individuals. Older persons spend 50% more on health care than they did in 1977. Out-of-pocket costs now exceed 19% of their income, *excluding long-term care.* These out-of-pocket expenses averaged $1,540 per older person in 1987 (Waldo, Sonnefeld, McKusick, & Arnett, 1989) and rose to $2,100 per older person in 1997 (American Association of Retired Persons [AARP] & Lewin Group, 1997). Out-of-pocket health care expenditures represent a significant burden on the elderly and are inversely related to their ability to pay for them. For older Medicare beneficiaries with incomes below the poverty line, out-of-pocket costs (excluding the costs of long-term care) are 35% of annual household income; for those at 100% to 125% of poverty, these costs are 23%; these costs make up 10% of annual household income for elders whose incomes are over 400% of poverty (AARP & Lewin Group, 1997). In addition, out-of-pocket costs for nursing home care are projected to rise significantly over time. In 1993, older nursing home residents, aged 65 to 84 spent more than 30% of their incomes for this care, and those 85 and older spent 40% (Komisar, Lambrew, & Feder, 1996). Over 50%

of women and one third of men who live to the age of 65 will spend some time in a nursing home, although one quarter of them will be there less than 3 months. Projections are that, in the future, patients will privately pay out of pocket a larger proportion of the costs of nursing home care between 2000 and 2030, resulting in a fivefold increase in U.S. total of out-of-pocket costs for nursing home services (rising from $33 billion or 31% of these costs to $158 billion or 48% of these costs) (American Council on Life Insurance [ACLI], 1998; Friedland & Summer, 1999). This is occurring in the context of the rise in total nursing home expenditures from $69 billion in 2000 to $330 billion in 2030 (ACLI, 1998; Friedland & Summer, 1999).

Other evidence of a "crisis" in health care has to do with the elderly as disproportionate users of health services (Evashwick, Rundall, & Goldiamond, 1985; Soldo & Manton, 1985). In the late 1980s, older persons made up just over 12% of the total U.S. population but accounted for more than 33% of health care expenditures (Waldo et al., 1989). Rice (personal communication, March 15, 2000) projects that in 2040, the elderly will be 20% of the population and account for 50% of the health care expenditures.

Changing Dependency Ratios

Alarm over disproportionate population growth of the aged and the social costs of their care has directed attention to the ratio of persons of working age (aged 20 to 64) to those not participating in the labor force (individuals under the age of 20 and the elderly aged 65 years and over). This ratio, called the "dependency ratio," or more recently the "support ratio," reflects the fact that goods and services allocated to those who are still in school or retired must be produced and supported by the working population. How much is available is conditioned by the size of the working population, its average productivity, the wage and price structure, and the willingness of its working members to assume taxes to finance the costs of supporting retired persons (Clark & Spengler, 1980; Taeuber, 1992).

Concern has been expressed over the increasing ratio of elders to those who are aged 20 to 64 years. As shown in Table 7.1, this ratio is expected to increase from approximately 21 per 100 in 1990 to 38 older persons per 100 persons working age (20-64) in 2050 (U.S. Bureau of the Census, 1993). However, the total dependency ratio (the number

Table 7.1   Elderly-to-Other-Adults Support Ratios, by Race and Hispanic Origin: 1990 and 2050

Race/Hispanic Origin	1990	2050
Total	21.3	38.2
White	22.7	42.9
Black	14.7	25.4
Other races[a]	9.9	26.6
Hispanic origin[b]	9.2	26.4

SOURCE: U.S. Bureau of the Census (1993).
NOTE: The elderly to working-age adults support ratio is the number of persons aged 65 years and over divided by the number of persons aged 20 to 64 × 100.
a. Includes Asian/Pacific Islanders, as well as American Indians, Eskimos, and Aleuts.
b. Persons of Hispanic origin may be of any race.

of youth and elders combined compared with the working population) will actually be *reduced,* when comparing the ratio for 1970 with those projected for 2000 and 2050. In other words, barring unforeseen events, there will be *fewer* dependents(under the age of 18 and aged 65 or older) per worker in the 21st century than there were between 1950 and 1970 (Brotman, 1982).

Of equal concern, is the two-elderly-generation ratio, the ratio for "two elderly generations" which is the number of persons aged 85 years and over per 100 persons aged 65 to 69 years (Siegel & Taeuber, 1986). Table 7.2 shows that in 1990, the overall ratio was 30 and similar for whites yet slightly lower among blacks. The ratio of 30 indicates that there were about three times as many persons aged 65 to 69 years as there were individuals aged 85 and over. The two-elderly-generation ratio is expected to increase steadily from 1990 to 2010. In the decades to follow, it would decrease somewhat until 2030, when a large number of individuals reach age 65 through 69 who are primarily in the baby boom generation. Interestingly, by 2050 the two-elderly-generation ratio will reach 100, indicating that there will be the exact number of persons aged 65 to 69 as there are individuals aged 85 and over. Simply

Table 7.2   Two-Elderly-Generation Support Ratio, by Race and Hispanic Origin: 1990 to 2050

Race/Hispanic Origin	1990	2010	2030	2050
Total	30	50	44	100
White	31	52	46	109
Black	26	35	26	57
Other races[a]	17	36	48	82
Hispanic origin[b]	21	39	37	84

SOURCE: U.S. Bureau of the Census (1993).
NOTE: The two-elderly-generation support ratio is the number of persons aged 85 years and over divided by the number of persons aged 65 to 69 years × 100.
a. Includes Asian/Pacific Islanders, as well as American Indians, Eskimos, and Aleuts.
b. Persons of Hispanic origin may be of any race.

stated, this means that many more older persons, particularly women in their late 60s, will have the added burden of caring for relatives, parents, and spouses in their mid-80s or older. This phenomenon will become more apparent for white Americans, with other racial/ethnic groups following closely behind, with the exception of blacks.

Economic and Social Well-Being

The economic status of the elderly has improved substantially over the past three decades. In fact, there is a general perception that the elderly are economically well off. Although the elderly today have achieved higher levels of economic security than earlier generations, one cannot infer that they are wealthy. To a large extent, the economic status of the elderly results from the accumulation or lack of accumulation of financial resources throughout one's lifetime. Differential rates are apparent in the general elderly population but also across certain subgroups, particularly among women, minorities, never-married, and widowed individuals.

Table 7.3   Median Income, by Age, Sex, and Marital Status, 1996

Sex and Marital Status	65-69	70-74	75-79	80-84	85 or older
Married couples	$32,988	$27,880	$24,655	$24,633	$23,373
Nonmarried men	15,101	14,313	14,106	13,025	10,928
Nonmarried women	11,630	11,325	10,294	10,171	9,417

SOURCE: Grad (1998).

Role of Age and Marital Status in Income Inequalities

In 1996, the median income of elderly individuals declined at every successive age grouping among men and women, irrespective of marital status (see Table 7.3). On the whole, married elders have median incomes nearly twice as high as nonmarried elders in each age group. However, Table 7.3 shows that for every age group among the elderly, nonmarried women have lower median incomes compared with nonmarried men or married couples. For example, nonmarried women between the ages of 75 and 79 earned only 73% of what men earned in the same age group. The gender gap is smallest among persons aged 85 and older, with women earning a median income 86% of that earned by men.

Role of Gender and Race/Ethnicity in Income Inequalities

In addition to income disparities by marital status within the elderly population, there is also considerable variation in economic status by race and ethnicity as well as by gender. As shown in Table 7.4, in 1998 whereas slightly over one third (36%) of elderly white women had incomes below $10,000, the proportion of blacks in this category is 71.0%, and for Hispanics, it is 76.5%. Among men, both blacks and Hispanics are more than twice as likely to fall into this low-income category compared with their white counterparts. This pattern is also evident for the second-lowest income category ($10,000 to $19,999). For the remaining four income brackets, ranging from moderate to high incomes, white men are more likely to fall into these categories than any other group. Minority elderly men and women as well as white

Table 7.4   Total Money Income of Nonmarried Individuals Aged 65 and Older: Percentage Distribution, by Sex, Race, and Hispanic Origin, 1998

	Less than $10,000	$10,000 to $19,999	$20,000 to $29,999	$30,000 to $49,999	$50,000 to $69,999	$70,000 or more	Median Income
				Women			
White	36.0	41.2	11.6	7.4	2.3	1.8	$12,097
Black	71.0	19.9	6.0	2.1	0.4	0.6	$7,629
Hispanic origin[a]	76.5	18.5	2.8	1.6	0.4	0.2	$6,954
				Men			
White	26.2	35.8	15.7	11.2	5.2	6.0	$15,812
Black	55.4	30.3	7.3	4.9	0.0	2.3	$9,449
Hispanic origin[a]	56.0	27.3	10.4	3.0	2.2	1.0	$9,279

SOURCE: U.S. Social Security Administration (1998b).
NOTE: Numbers may not add up to 100 due to rounding.
a. Persons of Hispanic origin may be of any race.

women are more likely to earn lower median incomes than are white men. Furthermore, the median income for white men is more than double that of elderly black and Hispanic elderly women ($15,812 vs. $7,629 and $6,954, respectively). White women have incomes at least 50% greater than those earned by both black and Hispanic elderly women. The racial/ethnic gap is also apparent among men. White men have a median income more than 67% greater than blacks and more than 70% greater than Hispanics.

Wide variability in income status by gender and racial/ethnic group membership is also reflected in poverty rates. As shown in Figure 7.2, white women are twice as likely as men to live in a family with income below the federal poverty threshold. Among black and Hispanic individuals aged 65 and older, women are 1.3 times more likely to be poor than men. Some argue that the large proportion of women who are widowed can account for the gender gap in poverty. Elderly women are particularly vulnerable to experiencing declines in their financial status as a result of losing a spouse (Bound, Duncan, Laren, & Oleinick,

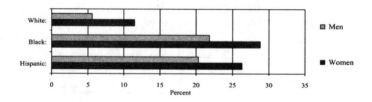

Race, Hispanic Origin, and Sex		Percentage
White		
	Women	11.5
	Men	5.6
Black		
	Women	28.8
	Men	21.8
Hispanic		
	Women	26.3
	Men	20.3

Figure 7.2. Percentage in Poverty Among Individuals Aged 65 and Older, by Sex, Race, and Hispanic Origin, 1997

SOURCE: Dalaker J., & Naifeh, M. U.S. Bureau of the Census, Poverty in the United States: 1997. Current Population Reports; Series P60-201. Washington, DC: U. S. Government Printing Office.

1991). It has been estimated that 80% of widows who are poor were not poor before they became widowed (Burkhauser & Smeeding, 1994).

As in the case of poverty, the proportion of the elderly population in "near poverty" or having incomes between the poverty line and 125% of the poverty line, is also likely to vary by race and ethnicity (Grad, 1998). In 1996, the near-poverty rate for whites was 9%. The rate for blacks and Hispanics was 25% and 24%, respectively. In 1997, the last year for which statistics are available, fully 17% of Americans aged 65 and older were poor or near poor as defined by the federal government, having annual incomes no higher than $9,623 (AARP & Lewin Group, 1997).

Thus far, the data have been presented on income for whites and racial and ethnic minorities. However, racial differences in income cannot fully explain the large racial disparity in wealth that exists today. According to Oliver and Shapiro (1995), although elderly blacks earn $2,380 less than whites, the wealth disadvantage among blacks is even more pronounced. By the time whites become senior citizens, they are

Table 7.5 Wealth, by Race, for Individuals Aged 64 and Older

	Black	White	Black/White Ratio
Income	$9,792	$12,172	0.76
Net worth	15,774	77,020	0.20
Median net financial assets	—	22,902	—
Mean net financial assets	6,640	71,510	0.09

SOURCE: Oliver and Shapiro (1995).

likely to have accumulated a net worth or net financial resources (all assets less any debts) that is nearly five times greater than black persons aged 64 or older (see Table 7.5).

Table 7.5 also shows that in contrast to net worth, the racial disadvantage between white and black elders for financial net assets is tenfold. The racial gap in wealth accumulation is largely due to blacks having less job security, fewer years of employment with a company, and a higher likelihood of encountering discrimination, which may lead to barriers in career advancement, creating a "glass ceiling" to better employment opportunities.

Social Class and Health

A considerable volume of research has consistently revealed that socioeconomic status (SES), whether measured by income, education, employment, occupation, poverty, or wealth, is one of the strongest known determinants of variations of morbidity and mortality in the general population (Adler, Boyce, Chesney, Folkman, & Syme, 1993; Antonovsky, 1967; Bunker, Gomby, & Kehrer, 1989; Williams, 1990). An inverse association between SES and mortality is found in early as well as recent reports and exists in virtually all countries where the association has been examined (Adler et al., 1994; Adler et al., 1993; Bunker et al., 1989; Feinstein, 1993; Feldman, Makuc, Kleinman, & Cornoni-Huntley, 1989; Haan, Kaplan, & Camacho, 1987; Krieger & Fee, 1994; Krieger, Rowley, Herman, Avery, & Phillips, 1993; Marmot,

Kogevinas, & Elston, 1987; Wilkinson, 1986). Feldman and colleagues (1989) found that mortality differences across educational groups exist for both men and women during the middle and older ages. Waitzman (1988) found a similar relationship for occupational status and mortality, particularly among men, that persisted throughout their later years.

In the past century, despite improvements in public health measures, standard of living, medical technology, and the delivery of and access to medical services, the socioeconomic differential between the wealthiest and the poorest has declined only slightly over time. For example, since the implementation of Great Britain's National Health Service, the health of all groups has improved. However, the highest socioeconomic groups have experienced a greater improvement in health status over time, such that the gap in health between high-SES groups and low-SES groups has not narrowed (Wilkinson, 1986).

SES status affects rates of chronic illness, disability, and death for all ages throughout the life course. However, differences in health by SES are smaller among the elderly when compared with younger individuals. Findings from the 1992 National Health Interview Survey (NHIS) show that poor elderly individuals are twice as likely as elderly with moderate or high incomes to report their health to be fair or poor (National Center for Health Statistics [NCHS], 1994). In addition, an inverse relationship between age-adjusted family income and limitations in activity due to chronic conditions was found among the aged (NCHS, 1994). As discussed in the preceding section, elderly minority individuals are far more likely than their white counterparts to have lower levels of SES. Recent research has found that SES predicts mortality variations for both blacks and whites. Rogot (1992), using the National Longitudinal Mortality Study (NLMS), documents that higher levels of both education and income predict lower rates of mortality. For example, it has been estimated that for African Americans and whites, the mortality ratios for individuals with a total family income of less than $5,000 (in 1980 dollars) were at least twice those of families with incomes of $50,000 or more (Rogot, 1992).

An alternative way of evaluating socioeconomic status in relation to health variation is to consider material and social conditions inherent in one's position in society. The Black Report, a seminal study conducted by researchers in the United Kingdom, emphasized the importance of area-based or aggregate measures of structural conditions—one's living and working environments—that predict variations in health

(Black, Townsend, & Davidson, 1982). In the United States, Haan and her colleagues (1987) found that residents of poor neighborhoods had a 70% higher rate of mortality than residents living in nonpoor neighborhoods. They concluded that living in poor neighborhoods is associated with adverse health outcomes as a result of poor housing conditions, high crime, and unmeasured factors in the social environment. More recent research has directed attention to understanding the conditions of the social environment, particularly residential characteristics, and its contribution to understanding variations in health (Collins & Williams, 1999; Krieger, Williams, & Moss, 1997; Robert, 1999; Yen & Kaplan, 1999; Yen & Syme, 1999). A provocative study by Collins and Williams (1999) found that living in racially segregated cities tends to be related to specific types of mortality for both black and white adults between the ages of 15 and 64 even after taking into consideration indicators of socioeconomic deprivation. It is well documented that blacks live in neighborhoods that are qualitatively different from whites. Both at the individual level (Williams & Collins, 1995) and ecological levels (Krivo & Peterson, 1996), poor black households are not comparable with white ones in terms of SES. For example, the extent to which widespread public housing is associated with high rates of crime is one factor that distinguishes poor black neighborhoods from those where whites live. In general, elders living alone tend to be more socially isolated. Future research is needed to understand how the "triple jeopardy"—the negative effects of age, racial/ethnic minority status, and low SES status—may affect the subjective well-being and other measures of health among the elderly. Other studies have directed attention to understanding both the community context and individual-level indicators of SES that may contribute to health outcomes across the life course (Robert, 1999).

Social Support and Health

The often-repeated finding of the importance of social networks and social support in physical and mental health is also striking. The evidence linking stress, illness, and social support dates back 50 years and includes the work of Berkman and colleagues (Berkman & Breslow, 1983; Berkman & Syme, 1979) and Lowenthal and Robinson (1976). More recent treatments of this issue (Pearlin, Aneshensel, Mullan, &

Whitlatch, 1996) and data consistent with earlier work are found in
Rowe and Kahn (1997, 1998), Kaplan and Haan (1989), and Ulbrich
and Bradsher (1993).

An important determinant of social support is the marital status of
older people. Widows and widowers are five times more likely than married persons to be institutionalized; elderly persons who never married
or have been divorced or separated have up to 10 times the rate of
institutionalization of married persons. In 1993, 9.4 million elders
lived alone, with the majority being women, 71% of which represent
white women 65 years of age or older (U.S. Bureau of the Census,
1994). In both 1988 and almost a decade later in 1997, the proportion
of older Americans living alone remained approximately one third of
the population (Commonwealth Fund, 1988). The proportion living
alone increases with age, with women aged 65 to 84 being twice as likely
as men to live alone. At age 85, 60% of women lived alone. Also among
persons 85 and older, men are four times as likely as women to live with
a spouse (NCHS, 1999b). Being single (widowed, divorced, or never
married) is highly associated with low income, particularly for women.
Persons experiencing the combination of living alone and having low
income have the highest risk of institutionalization (Butler & Newacheck,
1981; Commonwealth Fund, 1988).

Given that marital status and living arrangements are important
elements in understanding the health risks of the older population and
that living alone and being unmarried are seen as higher risks than not
living alone or being married, future projections concerning marital
status of the elderly are highly relevant to health. Work from the Urban
Institute (as reported by Steuerle, 1999) shows that there has been a
drastic change in marital status between 1970 and 1997. There has been
more than a threefold jump in the divorced category. The proportion
of married women dropped precipitously, from 81.4% to 67.9% in this
period. In 1997, one third of women were unmarried compared with
18.6% in 1970 (Estes & Michel, 1999).

Research on elderly minority individuals indicates that the proportions
of elderly blacks living alone (males, 23%; females, 37%) and American
Indians living alone (males, 20%; females, 35%) are similar. In comparison, the rates are 14% for males and 27% for females among Hispanic
elders (U.S. Bureau of the Census, 1994). The proportion of Asian/Pacific
Islander elders living alone is lower than all four racial/ethnic groups
(males, 8%; females, 16%). It is widely assumed that Hispanics live in

large, close-knit families, that they respect their elders, and that they place a high value of caring for them in their home. Cantor and Little (1985) suggest that it is not clear whether this is a factor of SES or culture distinctions. To a large extent, Asian Americans place a high value on the care of their elders. However, this trend has weakened in the past decade, and many Asian Americans are relying on formal care networks instead (Morioka-Douglas & Yeo, 1990). It has been well documented that African Americans tend to refer to extended informal social networks, such as family, friends, and the church as it relates to the care of their elders (Taylor & Chatters, 1991). There is little known about social support and Native Americans, given the limited availability of data among this population. However, it is well documented that the degree to which Native Americans are acculturated into mainstream society has weakened the position of the elderly American Indian. It is important to note that each of these groups is quite diverse and the heterogeneity that exists within each group should be examined in greater detail.

Scientific work has established both a theoretical basis and strong empirical evidence supporting the notion that social relationships affect health. In their review of this issue, House, Landis, and Umberson (1994) conclude that prospective studies, which control for baseline health status, consistently show increased risk of death among persons with a low quantity, and sometimes low quality, of social relationships. Experimental and quasi-experimental studies of humans and animals also suggest that social isolation is a major risk factor for mortality from widely varying causes.

The search for a mechanism that might explain why social support exerts so powerful an influence on health has generated a number of hypotheses. Most fall within one of two broad conceptual categories. The first, labeled the *direct* or *main effect* hypothesis, suggests that social support plays a health-promoting role regardless of stress level. The second, termed the *buffering* hypothesis, argues that social support works by protecting the individual from harmful psychological or physiological effects of stressful events (Ulbrich & Bradsher, 1993).

As researchers have struggled to specify and empirically test these notions, several important issues have arisen. First, what levels of "exposure" to social support (or, conversely, to social isolation) result in a health effect? Second, what are the differential effects, if any, of instrumental and expressive support? Third, which types of social relationships are supportive and which are harmful? Fourth, as

Minkler cautioned, what combinations of social support, intervention, and policies will ensure that social support will promote health (Minkler & Estes, 1991)?

Obviously, there is a great deal yet to be learned about social support and its effects on the health of the elderly population. Mechanic (1983) noted that much is unknown about the unique and joint effects of factors such as social class and social support on health. The effects of these social characteristics are interrelated, and rigorous studies are needed to separate confounded effects. In many instances, cause and effect are not clear, and the associations between variables and health status may reflect the fact that people with particular health characteristics systematically select themselves, or are selected, into certain social situations. Nevertheless, there appears to be sufficient evidence, especially with regard to difficulties encountered by elderly persons living alone, to warrant concern over the isolation and the lack of support that characterize the social situations in which many older Americans live.

The relationship between class and health, as described in the earlier section of this chapter, involves issues related to the etiology of disease and probability of death, to the access to treatment and the quality of care received, as well as to the differential occupational health risks that have direct and long-lasting influence on health status. The social and economic situations of elders, both past and current, are major determinants of their ability to maintain physical well-being and independence. On the whole, elders persist in the ability to have productive lives long after they are socially discredited from being able to do so.

Mortality

Life expectancy at birth has increased dramatically in the past 100 years, primarily as a result of substantial declines in mortality among infants. The expected number of years of life increased since 1900 for both men and women; however, women can expect to live longer than men, and whites are expected to live longer than their black counterparts. In 1996, life expectancy was approximately 5 years longer for white women than for black women and 7 years longer for white men compared with black men (see Table 7.6). Life expectancy also varies at older ages across racial groups.

Table 7.6. Life Expectancy at Birth, Age 65 and Age 85, by Sex and Race, 1996

Sex and Age	White	Black
Women		
At birth	79.7	74.2
At age 65	19.1	17.2
At age 85	6.3	6.2
Men		
At birth	73.9	66.1
At age 65	15.8	13.9
At age 85	5.3	5.3

SOURCE: Anderson (1998).

Table 7.6 shows that at age 65, the racial gap between blacks and whites persists but is much smaller than the black-white disparity in life expectancy at birth. Among elders who survive to age 65, white women would live an additional 19.1 years compared with 17.2 years for black women. White men at age 65 would survive 15.8 years compared with 13.9 years for black men. Among those who reach age 85, white women have the highest level of life expectancy. Interestingly, life expectancy at the oldest ages by race shows very little difference between the two groups. That is, the black life expectancy for both genders is similar to that observed for whites. This pattern is a departure from earlier data showing a "black-white crossover" in life expectancy at the oldest ages, with black life expectancy at age 85 exceeding the corresponding life expectancy for whites (Wing, Manton, Stallard, Hames, & Tryoler, 1985). Some researchers argue that blacks who reach the oldest ages may on average be healthier than white elders and have lower mortality rates (Manton, Stallard, & Wing, 1991). However, recent research by Preston, Elo, Rosenwaike, and Hill (1996) documents that the black-white crossover in mortality experience is largely the result of age misreporting at the oldest ages among blacks. Mortality statistics show that African Americans have a similar life expectancy to that of whites at the oldest ages simply because the majority of deaths among

Table 7.7. Number of Survivors, Out of 100,000 Persons Born Alive, Age 65 and Age 85, by Race and Sex, 1996

Sex and Age	White	Black
Women		
At age 65	86,918	76,405
At age 85	42,881	30,882
Men		
At age 65	77,887	59,819
At age 85	25,895	14,808

SOURCE: Anderson (1998).

blacks occur before they reach age 65, with the pattern being more pronounced among black men. Table 7.7 illustrates this point.

According to data for 1996, of a cohort of 100,000 black female babies, only 76% (76,405) reach the age of 65 compared with 86% (86,918) of white female births. Alternatively, 24% of black women died before reaching the age of 65 compared with 14% of white women. Only 59% of all black male infants survive to age 65 compared with 77% of all white male infants. In 1996, 86% of deaths for black men occurred before they reached the age of 85 compared with 75% of white men, 70% of black women, and 58% of white women.

In 1997, the overall death rate among those aged 65 and older was higher among men than women. Among individuals aged 65 to 74 and 75 to 84, mortality rates are highest among black women and men compared with other racial and ethnic groups (see Figure 7.3), Asians or Pacific Islanders and Hispanics have lower mortality rates than both black and white elders. Among persons aged 85 years and over, mortality rates are lowest for American Indian women. It is important to note that across all age mortality, statistics for the various racial and ethnic groups are subject to debate because of data inconsistencies that may either underestimate or overestimate mortality rates of these groups.

Deaths per 100,000 population

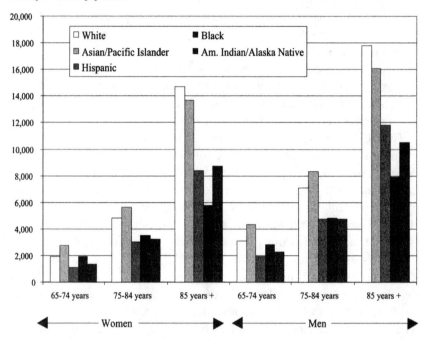

Figure 7.3. Death Rates for All Causes Among Individuals Aged 65 and Older, by Age, Sex, Race, and Hispanic Origin, 1997
SOURCE: U.S. Department of Health and Human Services (1999).

Morbidity

Morbidity is highly related to mortality, although the nature of their relationship in old age is debated. Fries (1980) postulates a biological limit for the human life span, arguing that as the limit on human life expectancy is approached, the onset of chronic disease will occur at ages closer to death; this will shorten the period between disease and death. Control over chronic disease through personal responsibility for disease prevention will diminish premature death so that people will live healthfully throughout most of their allotted 85 years, dying of senescence rather than disease; disease will be compressed toward the very end of life. Kramer (1980) and Gruenberg (1977) and others disagree with Fries, predicting that longer life spans will result from the control of the deadly outcomes of chronic disease, that people will live with chronic disease for more extended periods, and that the prevalence of morbidity in the population (the number of sick people at any given time) will be higher (Olshansky, Rudberg, Carnes, Cassel, & Brody, 1991; Rice & Feldman, 1983; Verbrugge, 1989). This will place even greater demands on the health system.

In addition to racial differences in life expectancy, there are racial differences in a variety of chronic conditions and activity limitations. Overall, the proportion of the elderly (aged 65 and older) with activity limitations is 38.5%, whereas the proportion of those aged 85 and older rises above half of the population (56.6%) (Disability Rights Advocates, 1997). There are limitations of activity due to chronic conditions for different racial and ethnic groups at older ages, including Asian/Pacific Islanders, blacks (non-Hispanic), white Hispanics, and whites. Health status according to this measure is poorest for older blacks, with only 35.6% reporting no activity limitations, compared with 43.6% of whites, 51.2% of white Hispanics, and 62.8% of Asian/Pacific Islanders (LaPlante & Carlson, 1996). Furthermore, having a lower income, having less education, and being a woman increase the risk of having higher rates of activity limitations due to chronic illness. In 1992, the proportion of those aged 65 and older without activity limitations is much higher (63.5%) for older persons with incomes above poverty and less than half for those elders below poverty (47.6%). A higher percentage of persons with activity limitations have lower educational levels compared with those with higher levels (LaPlante & Carlson, 1996). The most recent NHIS data (NCHS, 1999a) reveal that in 1996, fully 62% of those aged 70 and older had no activity limitations and that slightly more men than women reported this positive health condition (63.3% and 61.8%, respectively). Whites (62.6%) are more likely than blacks (59.8%) aged 70 and older to report no activity limitations; hence, blacks are more likely to report activity limitations due to chronic conditions and much more likely to report limitations in amount or kind of major activity (15.4% for blacks compared with 10.4% of whites) in 1996. Also in 1996, the inverse relationship persists between income and activity limitations at every income level. Among those aged 70 and older, those with incomes under $10,000 have a higher proportion reporting activity limitations than do those in

Table 7.8   Activity Limitations Due to Chronic Conditions, Age 70+, By Income, 1996

	Percentage With Limitations
Under $10,000	48.2%
$10,000-$19,000	40.8%
$20,000-34,000	32.2%
$35,000+	30.8%

SOURCE: National Center for Health Statistics (1999a, table 68).

higher income categories (see Table 7.8). Almost half (48.2%) of those in the lowest income category report activity limits (under $10,000), compared with 30.8% in the highest income category ($35,000 and higher) (NCHS, 1999a).

The presence of a disability is another indicator of some form of dependency. Using a broad definition of disability, data have been calculated for disability status and severe disability status for persons by age categories, demonstrating the increasing risk of disability with age. However, even among persons age 85 and over, about 15% are disability free and a larger percentage (about one third) are without severe disability. There are important differences in disability, by racial and ethnic status, income, education, and gender. Another important observation supporting the social construction of dependency thesis advanced in this chapter is the "increasing evidence of considerable plasticity in the functioning in old age, laying the grounds for disability prevention approaches" (Jette, 1996, p. 103).

Manton has suggested that the disease-free life span is increasing and that individual age-related disability occurs more rapidly and closer to death than cohort or cross-sectional data appear to suggest. Manton and his colleagues indicate that not only is the rate of aging highly variable among individuals but negative stereotyping of elderly persons seriously underestimates their ability to maintain functional capacity at older ages (Manton, 1982; Manton, Corder, & Stallard, 1993, 1997), based on research findings of a decline in disability rates of 1.3% a year for older persons between 1982 and 1994. Thus, there are 1.2 million fewer persons aged 65 and older with disabilities than there would have been if the disability rate had not declined over this period. Furthermore,

NHIS data for older people show no evidence of increased prevalence of disability over the past two decades (NCHS, 1999a).

Ken Manton (1982) also has argued that recent accretions in the life span among the very old belie assertions of a ceiling on potential life span. Between 1960 and 1978, life expectancy for white females at age 85 increased 2 years, and for nonwhite females, 4.5 years. Verbrugge (1989) has presented three scenarios that continue to shape population dynamics. In the tertiary prevention scenario, costly and heroic medical measures save many persons from the brink of death, prolonging their lives without influencing their principal illnesses. In the scenario of secondary prevention, fatal chronic diseases are controlled (i.e., there is lower case fatality), with the result that more people have disease for more years of their lives. This is the scenario of longer life but worsening health. The scenario of primary prevention is typified by lifestyle changes that diminish comorbidity and the chances of acquiring disease. Verbrugge projects that the cumulative result of these three scenarios is an increase in "population frailty" as "intrinsically nonrobust people stay in the living population" (Verbrugge, 1989, p. 30).

The point is that declining mortality rates and increased life expectancy do not, by definition, produce improved health. A longer life does not inevitably mean a healthier life. Rice and Feldman (1983) contend that two phenomena will occur simultaneously: There will be an increasing number and proportion of old people in quite good health up to the point of death *and* an increasing number and proportion with prolonged severe functional limitations.

One side of the mortality-morbidity debate (especially Manton's work) has been cited as cause for optimism about the projected general health condition of individual older people. Experts currently differ in opinions concerning the probability of future *additional* disability rate declines and their implications for public policy and health expenditures. Regardless of what happens with future disability rates, most concur that there is little evidence that health care costs will decrease. Instead, the weight of professional opinion is that it is much more plausible that future health expenditures will rise significantly, driven by both the absolute increases in the aging of the population and the numbers of the oldest old and the increasing biotechnological content of the medical-industrial complex.

Long-term care is a major component of the projected cost increases with the aging of America (Estes, Swan, & Associates, 1993; Friedland & Summer, 1999; see also Chapter 10). In 1995, long-term care expenditures topped $91 billion, of which the elderly paid the largest portion (about 40% or $36 billion) out of pocket. Of long-term care costs, 70% are for nursing homes (General Accounting Office [GAO], 1998). To these costs must be added the costs of informal (unpaid) long-term care provided primarily by women, which exceeds approximately $200 billion annually (1997 data) by very conservative estimates (Arno, Levine, & Memmott, 1999), as described in Chapter 6.

According to the GAO (1998), future predictions of the need for long-term care are uncertain, given the disagreement among scientists about whether or not there are (or will be) actual delays in the onset of illness with the increases in life expectancy. As the GAO report notes,

[some] predict that declining death rates may actually increase the need for long-term care if more people live to develop age-related disabling conditions or live longer with existing disabilities. Others argue that disability is becoming increasingly compressed into a shorter portion of the lifespan, decreasing the number of years long-term-care is needed. (GAO, 1998, p. 6)

In addition, there is uncertainty about long-term care cost projections because of the inability to predict what policy shifts will occur in Medicare and Medicaid coverage, as well as in private insurance. Both factors (assumptions about morbidity-mortality trends and policy shifts) explain varying estimates of those needing long-term care (from two to four times the present number of disabled older persons) and different projections of future health care expenditures vary (GAO, 1998).

Most experts concur that there will not be any slowing in future health care cost increases that have been projected to accompany demographic aging, which includes absolute increases in the numbers of older persons and the rapid growth in the population aged 85 and older. Furthermore, there is broad agreement that in the future there will be significant and increasing demands both on the health and long-term care systems and on informal caregivers (mostly women) who do more than three fourths of the work of long-term care.

Use of Health Care

Use of health care is another phenomenon affecting health that is highly associated with social class. Among those reporting poor or fair health, there are moderate differences in use rates by gender, income, and education. Although most elderly are eligible for Medicare, research has shown that more Medicare benefits are provided to the upper and middle classes and to whites than are provided to lower classes and to blacks (Davis, 1985). Inequities in Medicare benefits are associated with income, race, and region. In the southern region of the United States, where 56% of the nation's aged nonwhites reside, the disparities between white and nonwhite Medicare beneficiaries persist (Ruther & Dobson, 1981). Wennberg and Cooper (1997) and Skinner and Fisher (1997) have amply demonstrated significant variations in Medicare spending by region.

Furthermore, older members of the upper and middle classes can afford to supplement Medicare benefits with private health insurance, and they are better able to meet the increasing cost of copayments and deductibles under Medicare than are older members of the lower-income classes. The age-adjusted percentage of older persons who have private health insurance to supplement Medicare is actually declining, dropping from 78% to 70% between 1994 and 1997. The proportion of the elderly with only Medicare coverage increased from 13% to 21% (NCHS, 1999b). Older non-Hispanic whites are more likely to have private insurance to supplement their Medicare coverage than are Hispanic and black elderly (NCHS, 1999b). Lack of health insurance coverage has been shown to negatively influence health care use, as does family income, race, and ethnicity. For example, women over 50 below the poverty line were one third less likely than nonpoor women to receive mammography screening (NCHS, 1999b), which is an effective preventive service in reducing deaths from breast cancer.

Recent Medicare policy changes, particularly those in the Balanced Budget Act (BBA) of 1997 also have increased the hardship of out-of-pocket costs for the elderly under Medicare, particularly for low-income persons (Moon & Gage, 1997). For example, Medicare premiums will rise from 5% to 9% of annual incomes of the low-income elderly between 1997 and 2007. Other changes in the BBA of 1997 have been shown to negatively affect access to home care for the most ill and most economically disadvantaged (Medpac, 1999).

Conclusion

In short, wealth and its distribution in the nation enormously affect the capacity to maintain health. Wealth provides greater opportunities for rest, sound nutrition, education, emotional security, lack of stress, and status as well as greater capacity to have illness treated (Butler & Lewis, 1982). Certainly, the amount of disposable income available to older persons influences important individual choices concerning independence and well-being. For these reasons, it can be argued strongly that improving the income of older persons may be the most beneficial health policy strategy (Ball, 1981; McKinlay & McKinlay, 1977).

Despite the well-documented seriousness of the dependency needs of the elderly and the clear indication that the problems associated with them will only magnify in the future, there has been little policy response. The past decade produced a failed Clinton health reform plan, including the only major long-term care proposal for the elderly advanced by any president (Estes, Wiener, Goldberg, & Goldensen, 2000).

8 The Medical-Industrial Complex and the Aging Enterprise

Carroll L. Estes
Charlene Harrington
David N. Pellow

Understanding social policy and aging necessitates a critical examination of two overlapping and mutually reinforcing structural arrangements: the medical-industrial complex and the aging enterprise. It is not enough to look at the existence of a health care system promoted by capital interests. The role of the state in reinforcing and promoting market-driven delivery systems cannot be ignored. The complicated and conflicting relationship between capital and the state creates the dynamic nature of the medical-industrial complex and the aging enterprise.

The concept of the medical-industrial complex was first introduced in the 1971 book, *The American Health Empire* (Ehrenreich & Ehrenreich, 1971), a report from the consumer activist organization Health-PAC. The medical-industrial complex refers to the health industry, which is made up of multibillion dollar enterprises that include doctors,

AUTHORS' NOTE: Material in this chapter is adapted and expanded from "Medical-Industrial Complex," by C. L. Estes, C. Harrington, and D. Pellow. In *Encyclopedia of Sociology:* Vol 3, 2nd edition, edited by E. Borgatta and M. Borgatta (pp. 1818-1832). (New York: Macmillan, 2000). The authors acknowledge the contributions of the late Solomon Davis to an earlier publication on the medical-industrial complex, portions of which appear in revised and updated form in this chapter.

hospitals, nursing homes, insurance companies, drug manufacturers, hospital supply and equipment companies, real estate and construction businesses, health systems, consulting and accounting firms, and banks. As employed by the Ehrenreichs, the structure of the medical-industrial complex suggests that the primary function of the health care system is not the delivery of services but, rather, the pursuit of profits, with secondary functions of research and education.

Since that time, a number of authors have examined the medical-industrial complex: Navarro (1976); Relman (1980); Estes, Gerard, Zones, and Swan (1984); Wohl (1984); and McKinlay and Stoeckle (1994). Himmelstein and Woolhandler (1986) argue that health care facilitates profit making by (a) improving the productivity (health) of workers, (b) ideologically ensuring the social stability needed to support production and profit, and (c) providing major opportunities for investment and profit. Profit, the last function, is now the driving force as health care has fully established itself as central in capitalist production.

Arnold Relman (1980), Harvard medical professor and editor of the *New England Journal of Medicine,* was the first mainstream physician to write about the medical-industrial complex, observing that the corporatization of medicine is a challenge to physician authority, autonomy, and even legitimacy for the doctors who become health care industry owners. Ginzberg (1988) and others (Andrews, 1995; Estes et al., 1984; Himmelstein & Woolhandler, 1986) have written about the monetarization, corporatization, and proprietarization of "health" care. By the mid-1980s, the phrase "medical-industrial complex" was so well recognized that the book appearing with the title *The Medical-Industrial Complex* begins not with a definition but, rather, with "the story of the explosive growth of . . . corporate medicine" and focuses on "medical moguls," monopoly, and a prescription for profit (Wohl, 1984).

The "aging enterprise" is a closely related construct that was first introduced by Estes in 1979:

The term describes the congeries of programs, organizations, bureaucracies, interest groups, trade associations, providers, industries, and professionals that serve the aged in one capacity or another. Major components include physicians, hospitals, the Social Security Administration, the Administration on Aging, state and area agencies on aging, congressional committees on aging, as well as the nursing home and insurance industries. (p. 2)

Under this definition, the health-related components of the aging enterprise are located within the medical-industrial complex; however, the aging enterprise recognizes the role of the state and institutional action that extends beyond health and into all arenas of aging-related activities. Although acknowledging the substantial influence of the health care delivery system on how aging is produced, the aging enterprise focuses on the relationship between social policy and the condition and needs of the elderly across the board (Estes, 1993).

Different elements of several components of the aging enterprise, including Social Security and community-based long-term care, are considered in separate chapters of this book. The current chapter seeks to address the area of intersection between the medical-industrial complex and the aging enterprise—namely, the large health care delivery system that provides services to the elderly. Using multiple levels of the theoretical model of social policy and aging, this chapter explores in detail the role of the state in the promotion of capital. The inherent conflict between the promotion of profit and the ongoing legitimation of the state is discussed within the context of the failure of health care reform efforts.

The Health Care System

Although the health care industry has certainly contributed to improvements in the health status of the population, it has also strengthened and preserved the private sector and protected a plurality of vested interests. In U.S. society, the medical-industrial complex functions economically as a source of growth, profit accumulation, investment opportunity, and employment (Estes et al., 1984). It also contributes to the human capital needed for productivity and profit by preserving an able-bodied workforce whose work is not sapped by illness (Rodberg & Stevenson, 1977), although another interpretation suggests that private capital's stability is built on the appropriation of the working-class population's health (Navarro, 1976, 1982, 1995).

Structure of the Health Care Industry

Today's medical-industrial complex and aging enterprise consist of the following components: hospitals; nursing homes; physicians (salaried and fee-for-service); home health agencies; supply and equipment manufacturers; drug companies; insurance companies; managed care organizations (HMOs, PPOs, IPAs); specialized centers ("urgi," "surgi," dialysis); hospices; nurses and all other health care workers; administrators, marketers, lawyers, and planners; and research organizations. In addition to these entities, thousands of other organizations are developing long-term care (e.g., case management, respite care, homemaker/chore person, independent living center) and other services for the disabled and aging, including social services that have incorporated health care components, such as senior centers.

The Role of Capital and the Marketplace

Changes in the Structure of the Industry

There were a number of significant changes in the structure of the health care industry between the 1970s and 1990s, including (a) rapid growth and consolidation of the industry into larger organizations; (b) horizontal integration; (c) vertical integration; (d) change in ownership from government to private, nonprofit, and for-profit organizations; and (e) diversification and corporate restructuring (MacKinnon, 1982; Starr, 1982). These changes occurred across the different sectors, which are dominated by large hospital, insurance, and managed care organizations (see also Chapter 4).

Rapid Growth and Consolidation

Health care has long been moved from its cottage industry stage with small individual hospitals and solo physician practitioners to large corporate enterprises. Health care corporations are diverse and growing in terms of size and complexity. Hospitals are the largest sector of the health care industry, and although the growth rate in hospital expenditures was increasing rapidly, the number of community hospitals actually declined from 5,830 in 1980 to 5,194 in 1995 (−11%) (American Hospital Association [AHA], 1996) (see Table 8.1). The number of community hospital beds also began to decline in 1980 from 988,000 to 873,000 in 1995 (−12%) (AHA, 1996).

Table 8.1 Community Hospitals and Beds by Ownership, 1980, 1990, and 1995

	1980		1990		1995	
Type of Ownership	Hospitals	Beds*	Hospitals	Beds*	Hospitals	Beds*
Nonprofit	3,322 (57%)	692 (70%)	3,191 (60%)	657 (71%)	3,092 (60%)	610 (70%)
Investor owned	730 (13%)	87 (9%)	749 (14%)	101 (11%)	752 (14%)	106 (12%)
State and local government	1,778 (30%)	209 (21%)	1,444 (27%)	169 (18%)	1,350 (26%)	157 (18%)
Total	5,830	988	5,384	927	5,194	873

SOURCE: Adapted from American Hospital Association (1989, 1996).
NOTE: Excludes federal psychiatric tuberculosis and other hospitals.
* Scale 1,000 beds.

Nursing homes grew rapidly in numbers of facilities and beds after the passage of Medicaid and Medicare legislation. In 1996, there were 17,806 licensed nursing facilities with 1.82 million beds (Harrington et al., 1998). The number of facilities increased by 25% and the number of beds increased by 37% between 1978 and 1996. More recently, their overall growth has leveled off, so that growth is not keeping pace with the aging of the population (Harrington et al., 1998).

Relatively new and influential corporate forces in the health industry are the managed care organizations such as health maintenance organizations (HMOs), preferred provider organizations (PPOs), and independent practice associations (IPAs). There has been a large growth in HMOs, which provide health care services on the basis of fixed monthly charges per enrollee. In 1984, there were only 337 HMOs with 17 million enrollees. By 1988, there were 31 million members enrolled in 643 HMOs (InterStudy, 1989). The number of managed care enrollees grew to more than 50 million in 1996 and is expected to reach 100 million by the year 2002. Nearly 75% of U.S. workers with health insurance now receive that coverage through an HMO, a PPO, or a point-of-service plan (McNamee, 1997). There have been numerous rounds of mergers and acquisitions among HMOs, and some non-profit HMO corporations have established profit-making operations (Gallagher, 1999). (See Chapter 4, this volume, for more discussion.)

PPOs are modified HMOs that provide health care for lower costs when the enrollee uses participating providers who are paid on the basis of negotiated or discount rates (U.S. Department of Commerce [DOC], 1990). In 1988, there were about 620 PPOs with about 36 million members.

Private health insurance companies are also one of the largest sectors of the health industry. In 1988, the United States had over 1,000 for-profit, commercial, health insurers and 85 Blue Cross and Blue Shield plans (Feldstein, 1988). These private insurance organizations, along with HMOs, PPOs, and other third-party payers, paid for 32% ($348 billion of $1,092 billion) of the total expenditures in 1997 (Srinivasan, Levitt, & Lundy, 1998).

Physician practice patterns also changed rapidly between the 1970s and 1990s, moving toward larger partnerships and group practices. In 1969, 18% of physicians were in group practices (with three or more physicians), compared with 28% in 1984 (Andersen & Mullner, 1989). It is estimated that about 75% of all practicing physicians are part of at least one qualified HMO (U.S. DOC, 1990). Thus, physicians are moving toward larger and more complex forms of group practice. In addition, physicians are actively involved in the ownership and operation of many of the newer forms of HMOs, PPOs, IPAs, and other types of corporate health care activities (Iglehart, 1989; Relman, 1980).

Horizontal Integration

The major changes in corporate arrangements have been the development of multiorganizational systems through horizontal integration. The formation of multihospital systems has grown tremendously within the industry. Ermann and Gabel (1984) estimated that there were 202 multihospital systems controlling 1,405 hospitals and 293,000 beds in 1975 (or 24% of the hospitals and 31% of all beds). In 1997, there were 280 multihospital systems controlling 1,514 hospitals, and 543,588 beds (a ratio of 8:2). This represents a 39% increase in the number of multihospital systems, a small (7%) increase in the number of hospitals, and an 86% increase in the number of beds between 1975 and 1997.

Multihospital corporations are becoming consolidated, with large companies controlling the largest share of the overall hospital market. Most of the recent increase in these systems has been the result of

Table 8.2   Hospitals and Beds in Multihospital Health Care Systems, by Type of
Ownership and Control, 1997

Type of Ownership	Total Not-for-Profit		Investor-Owned		All Systems	
	Hospitals	Beds	Hospitals	Beds	Hospitals	Beds
Owned, leased, or sponsored	1,343 (53%)	309,216 (62%)	887 (35%)	119,466 (24%)	2,525 (100%)	501,724 (100%)
Contract managed	171 (36%)	12,901 (31%)	301 (64%)	28,963 (69%)	472 (100%)	41,864 (100%)
Total	1,514 (50%)	322,117 (59%)	1,188 (40%)	148,429 (27%)	2,997 (100%)	543,588 (100%)

SOURCE: Adapted from American Hospital Association (1997, table B3).

purchasing or leasing existing facilities and mergers of organizations rather than of the construction of new facilities (see Table 8.2).

Vertical Integration

Vertical integration involves the development of organizations with different levels and types of organizations and services. One such type of integration has involved the linkage of hospitals and HMO and/or insurance companies. For example, National Medical Enterprises owned hospitals, nursing homes, psychiatric hospitals, recovery centers, and rehabilitation hospitals (Federation of American Health Systems [FAHS], 1990). There has also been an increase in the number of academic medical center hospitals that have relationships with proprietary hospital firms (Berliner & Burlage, 1990). Many of the major investor-owned health care corporations are diversified, with many different types of health care operations.

Changes in Ownership

Between the 1970s and 1990s, the organizational side of health care witnessed a surge in the growth of both for-profit and not-for-profit health care delivery corporations, initially in hospitals and later extending to other types of health organizations. The ownership of hospitals shifted from public to nonprofit and for-profit organizations (see Table 8.1). The percentage of government-owned community hospitals dropped from 30% of the total community hospitals in 1980 to 26% in 1995, and the percentage of total beds declined from 21% to 18% during the same period (AHA, 1996). In contrast, the percentage of proprietary facilities increased from 13% to 14%, and the percentage of proprietary beds increased from 9% to 12%, of the total during the 1980 through 1995 period. The percentage of total U.S. hospitals owned by nonprofit corporations increased from 57% to 60% during the period, but the percentage of beds remained at 70% (AHA, 1996). Of the total 280 multihospital systems in 1997 (down from 303 systems in 1988), investor-owned systems controlled 40% of the hospitals and 27% of the beds, compared with nonprofit facilities (AHA, 1997). The federal government controlled 9.8% of hospitals and 13% of beds, whereas nonprofit organizations controlled 50% of hospitals and 59% of beds (AHA, 1997). We note that this represents a 3% decrease in the number of hospitals and a 6% decrease in the number of beds in multi-hospital systems controlled by investor-owned systems since 1988.

Nursing homes have the largest share of proprietary ownership in the health field (except for the drug and medical supply industries). In 1997, approximately 65% of all nursing homes were profit making, 28% were nonprofit, and 7% were government run (Harrington, Carrillo, Thollaug, & Summers, 1999). By 1997, chains owned 54% of the total nursing home facilities.

For-profit companies dominate the HMO market. Between 1981 and 1997, for-profit HMOs grew from representing 12% to 62% of total HMO enrollees and from 18% to 75% of health plans (Srinivasan et al., 1998). Investor-owned corporations have also established themselves in many other areas of health care, ranging from primary care clinics to specialized referral centers and home health care. The number of proprietary home health corporations is increasing rapidly, but the number of traditional visiting nurse associations is declining (Estes, Swan, Bergthold, & Spohn, 1992). In 1982, it was estimated that 14% of the Medicare home health charges were by proprietary agencies, 26% by nonprofit organizations, 32% by visiting nurse associations, 15% by facility-based agencies, and 14% by other agencies (U.S. Department of Health and Human Services [DHHS], 1989). By 1996, proprietary agencies accounted for 44% of total Medicare agencies, nonprofit care for 37%, and government and others for 19% (U.S. DHHS, 1997).

Of home health agencies, 44% were part of a multifacility chain. This represents a dramatic shift in ownership within a 5-year period. The changes brought about by the for-profit chains are more extensive than their proportionate representation among health care providers might suggest (Bergthold, Estes, & Villanueva, 1990; Estes & Swan, 1994). By force of example and direct competition, for-profit chains have encouraged many nonprofit hospitals and other health entities to combine into chains and convert to for-profit status (Dube, 1999).

Diversification, Restructuring, and Growth

Diversification of health care corporations is continuing to occur. Some large hospital corporations have developed ambulatory care centers (such as Humana, which later sold its centers), whereas others have developed their own HMOs or insurance. By the mid-1980s, many experts expected America's health care system to be dominated by the four largest for-profit hospital chains: Hospital Corporations of America (HCA), Humana, National Medical Enterprises, and American Medical International. By the late 1990s, only Humana and HCA remained, and HCA had already merged with Columbia. Eventually, HCA Columbia almost collapsed as the result of a scandal over fraud during the late 1990s ("Blowing the Whistle," 1998). Economic problems in the late 1980s resulted in some industry restructuring, by scaling down operations and spinning off substantial segments (Ginzberg, 1988).

In the 1990s, this cycle repeated itself, as the frenzy of mergers and acquisitions has produced ever-greater desires for cost cutting and restructuring. One report states that much of the drive for cost containment stemmed from drug companies raising prices and an increase in patient visits to doctors (use costs) (Hayes, 1998). High stock values and the desire to improve market share have catalyzed many health care firms to seek growth through mergers and acquisitions. The number of mergers among health services (483) and HMO companies (33) peaked in 1996. These mergers were valued at $27 billion and $13.3 billion, respectively (Hayes, 1998).

As HMOs grow, it has become clear that their primary goals are market control, profit making, and cost containment (through capitation and other mechanisms). In the years 1994 through 1999, a dozen companies were merged or acquired by six of the biggest firms: Aetna,

Cigna, United Healthcare, Foundation Health Systems, PacifiCare, and WellPoint Health Networks. One example of a merger between Aetna and U.S. Healthcare in 1996 put a "corporate giant in control of the care of 1 in 12 people in the United States" (Slaughter, 1997, p. 22).

As managed care organizations became the dominant player in the health care industry in the 1990s, both doctors and patients began to voice complaints about the system. Many patients felt that they were no longer able to receive the quality time and personal care of a primary physician, because the latter were hurried through panels of patients to maintain efficiencies demanded by HMOs. For their part, many doctors argued that capitation and other structures introduced by HMOs limited their freedom to make treatment decisions. Many doctors and patients argued that these trends were producing lower-quality care (Fruedenheim, 1999). Additionally, registered nurses were increasingly being used in place of doctors to lower labor costs. Registered nurses, in turn, were also being replaced with less skilled and lower-paid personnel. In response, both doctors and nurses have begun a fervent effort to unionize (Slaughter, 1997). Although some critics argue that the impacts of this growth at all costs by both for-profit and nonprofit organizations are often devastating to communities (Bond & Weissman, 1997; Kassirer, 1997), others find few negative effects (Fubini & Stephanie, 1997).

Financial Status and Profits

The private health sector was marked by great volatility and growth in the 1990s. The *Forbes* annual report on investor-owned health corporations shows that median 5-year average return on equity for health corporations was 14.6%, well above the 10.5% for all U.S. industries (Condon, 1998) (see Table 8.3). Median health industry sales for investor-owned companies grew 8.8% for 1997 and at an 11.1% rate for the 5-year average. Earnings per share were 15.5% in the most recent 12 months, compared with 8.6% for the 5-year average. The earnings per share were higher than the 14.9% earnings for all U.S. industries in the most recent 12 months in 1997 (Condon, 1998).

The *Forbes* financial reports for the largest health corporations are shown in Table 8.3 for three different sectors of the industry: health care services, drugs, and medical supply companies (Condon, 1998; Hayes, 1998). The most profitable health care service corporation in 1989 was Humana, which owns both hospitals and insurance companies.

Table 8.3   Selected U.S. Health Care Investor Corporations, 1998

	Profitability Growth						Net Income
	Return on Capital		Sales		Earnings per Share		Income
	5-Yr. Avg.	Latest 12 Mo.	5-Yr. Avg.	Latest 12 Mo.	5-Yr. Avg.	Latest 12 Mo.	Latest 12 Mo.
Health care services	%	%	%	%	%	%	$ mil
Oxford Health Plans	36.5	4.2	116.0	46.2	74.7	−72.0	25
Mid Atlantic	34.4	2.7	21.7	2.9	NM	−67.6	5
Health Mgt.	20.8	22.3	25.0	25.4	33.2	27.6	108
WellPoint Health	19.8	15.0	15.1	43.0	6.0	17.2	203
Sun Healthcare	18.9[a]	7.4	89.9	28.2	NM	D-P	49
PacifiCare Health	18.3	18.2	33.7	69.5	8.9	37.0	124
United HealthCare	17.4	10.0	62.2	19.0	24.2	64.1	436
HBO & Co.	17.0	23.6	35.8	43.0	NM	63.6	145
Quorum Health	14.5	11.3	50.3	28.4	32.1	20.0	88
Humana	12.3	11.0	22.2	15.3	32.7	270.8	147
Medians	10.4	7.4	24.9	22.3	6.0	23.5	52
Drugs	%	%	%	%	%	%	$ mil
Schering-Plough	49.6	58.1	8.9	15.9	15.1	17.5	1,378
Abbott Labs	38.1	35.2	9.5	10.8	13.3	12.8	2,038
Amgen	35.4	29.6	25.1	10.6	37.4	0.9	643
Bristol-Myers Squibb	34.9	41.8	6.4	10.2	3.6	57.4	3,119
Warner-Lambert	32.1	19.7	7.6	6.2	32.5	8.6	805
Medians	14.3	11.7	14.7	10.7	11.9	15.8	198
Medical supplies	%	%	%	%	%	%	$ mil
Medtronic	28.1	31.5	16.5	8.7	27.2	15.5	564
Johnson & Johnson	26.5	26.2	11.5	7.3	14.6	14.7	3,229
Patterson Dental	24.4	20.4	18.9	19.9	30.6	24.3	37
Stryker	20.1	16.2	20.7	8.8	24.2	21.0	119
Perkin-Elmer	19.7	26.9	5.4	10.5	13.6	271.9	107
Medians	14.6	13.4	8.7	5.9	4.7	15.5	79
Industry medians	14.6	12.7	11.1	8.8	8.6	15.5	107
All Industry Medians	10.5	10.3	8.9	7.9	6.7	14.9	96

SOURCE: Adapted from Condon (1998).
NOTE: D-P = deficit to profit; NM = not meaningful.
a. Four-year average.

In 1989, its group health insurance division had almost 1 million members and a $4 billion operating profit (Fritz, 1990). The most profitable health care service corporation in 1997 was HBO & Company, and Oxford Health Plans had the strongest 5-year average.

Although large investor-owned HMOs are growing each year, the 1990s were tumultuous financially. As the *Forbes* annual report on American Industry put it, "Healthcare providers are supposed to make people well, but many of these companies are very sick themselves" (Hayes, 1998, p. 180). Although Oxford Health Plans had the higher 5-year average, from July 1997 to January 1998 its stock lost over 80% of its value. Similarly, the number-two ranked company, Mid Atlantic Medical Services, saw its stock drop by more than 50% of its value in a single year's time. Rapid growth, through mergers, acquisitions, and internal sales, "eventually outstripped management's ability to run these companies" (Hayes, 1998, p. 180).

Earnings per share of drug companies were at 15.8% in 1997, which was up from the 5-year average of 11.9% (Condon, 1998). Return on equity reported for drug companies was at 11.7% in 1997, significantly less than the 14.3% on average over the previous 5 years (Condon, 1998). On the other hand, earnings per share of medical supply companies were doing well at 15.5% in 1997, far better than their 5-year median earning of 4.7%. In 1989, a number of large drug company mergers occurred, particularly between U.S. firms and foreign corporations such as Genentech, Inc., and Roche Holding, Ltd., of Switzerland (Southwick, 1990). These international mergers continued into the 1990s.

Although the biotechnology industry did not show overall profits in 1989, the sales growth rates were strong, and some companies had high profit rates, such as Diagnostic Products, with a 22.3% earnings per share and 23.6% return on equity in 1989 over the previous year (Clements, 1990). Biotechnology saw an upsurge of economic growth and media coverage when several new developments emerged in the 1990s. The first was the introduction of "gene therapies" whereby scientists could modify a person's genetic makeup to fight against otherwise deadly or incurable diseases such as cancer and Alzheimer's. The second was the launching of the Human Genome Project, a massive effort by scientists in government and industry to "map" the structure of the human genetic code. The third, was the announcement, by a Scottish scientist in 1997, that he had successfully cloned a sheep from another sheep's DNA.

Although all of these developments signaled the importance of biotechnology in the future of health care research and policy, some observers were critical of these technological "advances." First, the cloning of animals such as sheep leaves open the distinct possibility that human beings might soon be cloned. The prospect of this event raised dire concerns among bioethicists, politicians, scientists, and religious leaders during 1997, and President Clinton issued a worldwide call to scientists to voluntarily refrain from such activities. Second, some critics have noted that the Human Genome Project has been associated with efforts to "locate" not only genes believed to be the cause of certain diseases such as breast cancer but also those genes believed to be associated with certain types of deviant, or criminal, behavior. Focusing on the genetic "causes" of certain diseases and social behaviors raises many problematic scenarios for public policy (e.g., defining criminal behavior as genetically based rather than being rooted in social structures). Third and finally, some biotechnology companies have been associated with efforts to patent life forms around the globe, including parts of the human body—prompting some critics to label this practice "biopiracy" or "biocolonization" (Kimbrell, 1996). Taken together, these charges suggest that, through biotechnology, the medical-industrial complex is charting revolutionary territory that has allowed private interests to define, claim ownership over, and even create life on this planet. Despite these criticisms, biotechnology stocks continue to rise. As noted, the pharmaceutical industry alone traded upward of $110 billion globally in 1997, and the overall U.S. health expenditures topped 1 trillion dollars by the end of the 1990s. Some analysts project health costs to more than double by 2015 to $2.3 trillion, of which the government share will be between 25% and 50% (Pardes et al., 1999).

In summary, the 1970s, 1980s, and 1990s were decades of enormous growth in health care spending and the rationalization of health care service delivery, with the formation of large, complex, bureaucratically interconnected units and arrangements that reached well beyond the hospital and permeated virtually all sectors of the health industry. At the same time, new sectors emerged (e.g., genetic research and subacute care), bringing additional industry developments. This vertical and horizontal integration of medical organizations and industries, combined with the revival of market ideologies and government policies promoting competition and deregulation, has profoundly altered the shape of U.S. health care delivery. In the 21st century, these changes continue to signal a fundamental social transformation of American medicine and a rationalization of the system under private control (Starr, 1982).

The Role of the State

The Need for Regulation

The federal government has been playing and continues to play a crucial role in the development of the medical-industrial complex. After World War II, the federal role expanded as Congress enacted legislation and authorized money for research, education, training, and the financing of health services. The passage of Medicare and Medicaid in 1965 was pivotal in expanding the medical-industrial complex and the aging enterprise as government became the third-party payer for health care services (Estes et al., 1984). As a consequence, public demand for health care among the aged, blind, disabled, and poor (all previously limited in access) was secure. Medicare and Medicaid provided the major sources of long-term capital financing for hospitals and contributed to the marked increase in service volume and technology, as well as to the continued oversupply of physicians (McKinlay & Stoeckle, 1994). Thus, federal financing of health care has performed the very important functions of sustaining aggregate demand through health insurance programs, protecting against financial risks, subsidizing research and guaranteeing substantial financial returns, supporting the system's infrastructure through training subsidies and capital expansion, and regulating competition through licensure and accreditation (LeRoy, 1979).

In the 1980s and 1990s, two other forces were responsible for the dramatic changes in the medical-industrial complex and aging enterprise: (a) a change in the ideological climate with the election of Presidents Reagan, Bush, and Clinton; and (b) changes in state policies to promote privatization, rationalization, and competition in health care (Estes, 1991b). These changes contributed to increases in the proportion of services provided by proprietary institutions (Schlesinger, Marmor, & Smithey, 1987). Although policies of the 1960s and 1970s encouraged a form of privatization built on the voluntary sector (Estes & Bergthold, 1989), Presidents Reagan and Bush shifted the direction and accelerated privatization. President Clinton introduced a Health Care Reform plan in 1993 that ultimately failed, giving way to a private sector-driven market reform managed care, promoting a system that many contend benefits investors over patients, doctors, and community hospitals (Andrews, 1995).

In the 1980s and 1990s, the form of privatization was government subsidy of a growing proportion of for-profit (rather than nonprofit) enterprises (Bergthold et al., 1990). There was also privatization in the form of a transfer of work from the formal sector of the hospital to the informal sector of home and family with ambulatory surgery and shortened lengths of hospital stays (Binney, Estes, & Humphers, 1993) promoted through government action. Regulatory and legislative devices were important in stimulating and accelerating privatization in the health and social services. The Omnibus Reconciliation Act of 1980 and the Omnibus Budget Reconciliation Act of 1981 contributed to competition and deregulation, private contracting, and growth of for-profits in service areas that were traditionally dominated by nonprofit or public providers (e.g., home health care). For-profit entities have nonprofit subsidiaries, and vice versa, and conceptual and structural complexities have multiplied, rendering impossible the simple differentiation of public from private. It is noteworthy that government-initiated privatization strategies did not reduce public sector costs.

Given the long-term historical role of the private, nonprofit sector in U.S. health and social services since the earliest days of the republic and the rapid organizational changes of the 1980s and 1990s, vertical and horizontal integration have blurred boundaries between the nonprofit and for-profit health care sectors (see Chapter 4). The distinction between for-profit and nonprofit is less meaningful when both organizational forms appear to be pursuing greater revenues through cost cutting and mergers. Eight of the 10 largest health care systems (by net patient revenues) in 1997 were nonprofits (Bellandi & Jaspen, 1998). That same year, 4 of the 10 largest health care systems (by number of hospitals owned) were also nonprofits (Bellandi & Jaspen, 1998). Whether nonprofits are oriented toward the needs of the community any more than for-profits is unclear, because many of these organizations (both insurance plans and hospitals) are undergoing "conversions" to for-profit status (Marsteller, Bovbjerg, & Nichols, 1998).

The concern that many communities have is that these conversions may mean less attention to the health needs of local residents. The increase in conversions has "heightened the need for accountability regarding the accurate determination and disposition of assets developed with the assistance of tax subsidies for nonprofit medical entities such as Blue Cross" (Estes & Linkins, 1997, p. 436). Federal and state laws require that their assets remain in the charitable sector and continue to be used for the community's benefit. Twenty-three states now have conversion laws clarifying the authority of attorney generals to regulate these conversions. Conversion laws mandate varying degrees of public participation and public disclosure but often are best implemented when there is an active community-based activist presence to monitor the organization's practices.

From social movements to the federal government, institutions across the nation are recognizing the increasing need for monitoring and regulation of the myriad branches of the medical-industrial complex. As noted earlier, physicians are advocating new legislation and even beginning to unionize against HMOs. Unfortunately, often when regulation exists, it is easily circumvented. For example, the Health Insurance Portability and Accountability Act of 1996 was intended to protect Americans who change or lose their jobs by ensuring portability of plans across groups and into the individual market. It was also intended to protect people against denial of coverage for preexisting conditions. However, many insurers have skirted this law by denying commissions to their agents who sell insurance to people with medical problems (Pear, 1997).

In other cases, there is little-to-no regulation of purchasers, such as large employers who self-insure under the Employment Retirement Income Security Act (ERISA) of 1974. These employers are exempt from state insurance laws and are bound by no federal regulation in this area. More than 125 million Americans who have HMO coverage cannot sue their provider for punitive damages. As *Time* magazine recently reported, this represents a clear subordination to corporate interests (Howe, 1999). Furthermore, the continuing rapid pace of mergers and acquisitions in the health care industry has created the consolidation of markets that raise questions about the need for antitrust policies directed at this sector.

At the federal level, the President's Advisory Commission on Consumer Protection and Quality in the Health Care Industry has called for a "consumer bill of rights," and others clamor for a "patient's bill of rights." These proposals would provide, for example, the right to sue HMOs for damages, prohibitions against negative financial incentives, and external reviews of patient complaints. Whether this proposal will ever become national legislation is unclear. But as the "new federalism" or previously federal responsibilities are "devolved" to the states, it is certain that 50 separate governments will have great difficulty coherently regulating a health care system for the entire nation. This is especially troublesome for the growing numbers of persons among the uninsured and those in need of long-term care (Estes & Linkins, 1997).

Long-term care is an area of health policy in need of greater attention as the age distribution of the population changes so that the number of persons over the age of 65 and over the age of 85 is increasing rapidly (see Chapter 10). Medicare, Social Security, and other entitlement programs affecting the elderly have been the focus of the "devolution revolution" (Estes & Linkins, 1997), which raises serious questions about the quality and accessibility of long-term care under managed care. There are profits to be made in this sector of the industry as well. One publication referred to 1997 as the "year of assisted living" because 7 of the top 10 health care provider organizations were assisted living companies and half posted returns of 50% or greater ("The Public Market," 1998). Long-term care will have to meet the "bottom-line" criteria of "cost saving" or "profit generation," and this is likely to produce problems for those in need of these services. Indeed, the needs of all less powerful groups—the elderly, the poor, the working and middle classes, women, and people of color—are increasingly being obscured by these business directives as well. Regulation of health care institutions in the interests of these marginalized groups is especially difficult when the American Medical Association is second to none in money spent on lobbying the Congress and state legislatures (Jaspen, 1999).

The U.S. Medical-Industrial Complex in a Global Context

The U.S. health care system ranks near the bottom of all industrialized nations on a number of key dimensions. The health of U.S. citizens is poorer and the number of under- and uninsured individuals is greater than any other industrialized nation. Among the top 24 industrialized nations, the U.S. ranks 16th in life expectancy for women,

17th in life expectancy for men, and 21st in infant mortality (Andrews, 1995). A Harris poll indicated that the citizens of Canada, Western Europe, the United Kingdom, and Japan report much higher satisfaction ratings for their health care system than do Americans (Isaacson, 1993). In contrast, compared with other nations, doctors in the United States receive much higher incomes relative to the average worker. For example, in 1987 the income ratio of doctors to the average worker in the United States was 5.4, whereas in Canada it was 3.7, and in Japan and the United Kingdom it was 2.4 (Isaacson, 1993). Thus, the poor performance of the United States on health indicators is ironic given that the United States spends more money on its health care system than any other nation in the world.

Because of the pluralistically financed health care system in the United States, administrative costs are much higher than those of the national and publicly financed health care systems of virtually all other Western industrialized nations, with the exception of South Africa. U.S. health care expenditures were increasing at an alarming rate until around 1993, when the rate of growth in expenditures began to slow. However, this trend is expected to reverse itself, and one study projects that health spending is expected to rise as a share of gross domestic product (GDP), climbing to an estimated 16.6% by 2007 (Smith, Freeland, Heffler, McKusick, & the Health Expenditures Projection Team, 1998).

Multinational health enterprises are an increasingly important part of the medical-industrial complex, with investor-owned and investor-operated companies active not only in the United States but also in many foreign countries. In 1990, a report showed 97 companies reporting ownership or operation of 1,492 hospitals with 182,644 beds in the United States and 100 hospitals with 11,974 beds in foreign countries (FAHS, 1990). The four largest for-profit chains owned two thirds of the foreign hospitals (Berliner & Regan, 1990). Pharmaceutical firms have also become major global corporate players. In 1990, foreign control over pharmaceutical production was 72% in Australia, 61% in the United Kingdom, 57% in Italy, and 30% in the United States (Tarabusi & Vickery, 1998). The total value of global pharmaceutical exports and imports is estimated to be in excess of $110 billion (Tarabusi & Vickery, 1998). The effects of these developments in foreign countries and the profit potential of these operations are not clearly understood (Berliner & Regan, 1990).

Examining the U.S. medical-industrial complex in a comparative context provides an understanding of the role of the welfare state and government vis-à-vis civil society and private capital. What has become clear is that the unique problems created by the U.S. medical-industrial complex are rooted in the subordination of the state and civil society to corporate interests. Other nations whose health care systems are much more effective are marked by the state's taking an active role to restrict the profit motive in health insurance, "or they simply never let a commercial market develop" (Andrews, 1995, p. 36). This is because voluntary insurance in many other countries historically preceded public legislation, and these insurance funds were linked to labor unions, political groups, and religious groups—not to private companies and health care providers, as in the United States. In these cases, government policy was, and remains, heavily influenced by nongovernmental organizations (NGOs)—namely, religious and labor groups. The medical-industrial complex in particular and corporate-civil society relations in general in the United States are much less democratic largely because of the lower levels of mobilization by trade unions and other NGOs. Government agencies in the United States can learn from other nations and begin to implement policies that leverage the power of the state and NGOs in ways that bring a greater balance among the stakeholders in the medical-industrial complex.

Conclusion

Commodification, commercialization, proprietarization, and *monetarization* are all terms used to describe the medical-industrial complex and aging enterprise dynamic: the potentially distorting effects of money, profit, and market rationality as a (if not the) central determining force. After three decades devoted to market rhetoric, cost containment, and stunning organizational rationalization, the net result is the complete failure of any of these efforts to stem the swelling tide of problems of access and cost. For example, although national health care expenditures make up around 15% of the GDP, the number of uninsured Americans was fully 43.4 million, or 16.1% of the population in 1997—the highest level in a decade (Kuttner, 1999). Moreover, there are alarming increases in the uninsured population among African Americans, Latinos, and the middle class (Carrasquillo, Himmelstein,

Woolhandler, & Bor, 1999). Of those Americans who do have insurance, a recent study found that the number of persons insured by the private sector is much less than previously believed. Whereas many studies had estimated that 61% of the insured received coverage through the private sector, Carrasquillo et al. (1999) found that the public sector subsidizes much of this coverage so that, in fact, only 43% of the population receives insurance through the private sector. Thus, not only is the burden on the state greater than previously thought because of this subsidy to the private sector, but the general decline in private insurance coverage will also produce further strains on the government's budget.

The rapidly growing health care industry is creating strains on the economic system while it also is creating a financial burden on government, business, and individuals through their payments for health services. Responses to these deficit strains and fluctuations have included cutbacks in services and reimbursements, cost shifts onto consumers, and alterations in the structure of the health care system itself to accord better with a competitive, for-profit model. The competition model as a prescription for the nation's health care woes has restricted access to health care and raised questions of quality of care (Bond & Weissman, 1997; Harrington, 1996; Kassirer, 1997). Cost shifting to consumers is increasingly limiting access to needed services for those with less ability to pay. Managed care has not delivered the cost savings it promised, and the Health Care Financing Administration acknowledges that Medicare does not benefit from cost reductions from HMO enrollment of elders due to continuing adverse risk selection (DePearl, 1999). Ironically, these responses are occurring simultaneously when, in 1999, a huge federal deficit has been turned into a surplus, an event of historic significance. The budget surplus has produced a combination of euphoria and vigorous debate over what the government should do with it. This surplus emerged against the backdrop of an unusually high economic growth rate and a strong U.S. economy in general.

Investor-owned health care enterprises have elicited a number of specific criticisms. It has been argued that commercial considerations can undermine the responsibility of doctors toward their patients and lead to unnecessary tests and procedures and, given other financial incentives, to inadequate treatment. The interrelationships between physicians and the private health care sector, particularly for-profit corporations, raise many issues about the effects on quality of care and health care use and expenditures. Many have argued that the potential for abuse, exploitation, unethical practices, and disregard of fiduciary responsibilities to patients is pervasive (Iglehart, 1989). Legislation has even been introduced in Congress that would prohibit physicians from referring patients to entities in which they hold a financial interest and from receiving compensation from entities to which they refer patients (Iglehart, 1989). At the end of the Clinton presidency, several versions of a "patient's bill of rights" remained at the center of bipartisan controversy at both the state and federal levels of government.

Critics of for-profits argue that such ownership drives up the cost of health care, reduces quality, neglects teaching and research, and excludes those who cannot pay for treatment. Opponents of the market model for health care reflect diverse interests, including members of the medical profession seeking to preserve their professional autonomy, advocates for access to health care for the poor and uninsured, those concerned about the impact of profit seeking on quality of care, and many others. As government and business attempt to restrain health care spending, cutting into profits and forcing cost reductions, public concerns intensify.

9 A Political Economy Critique of "Productive Aging"

Carroll L. Estes
Jane L. Mahakian
Tracy A. Weitz

Gerontologists have recently engaged in serious attempts to "reconstruct" the reality of aging—first from what is "usual" to what is "successful" and, now, from aging as a negative value (i.e., as "unproductive") to something valued (i.e., as "productive"). Recent work in gerontology has produced the theory of "productive aging" as a framework for the promotion of health, specifically in relation to the conditions and processes of aging. Productive aging attempts to counteract negative associations linked with the experience of aging and the status of the elderly, by focusing on the value of achievements and contributions made by aging individuals. This chapter offers a critique of "productive aging" that begins with a historical look at the ideological context of efforts to promote health in aging. Using multiple levels of the theoretical model advanced in Chapter 1, consideration is given to

AUTHORS' NOTE: Material in this chapter is adapted and revised from "The Political Economy of Productive Aging," by C. L. Estes and J. Mahakian. In *Productive Aging: Concepts and Challenges*, edited by N. Morrow-Howell, J. Hinterlong, & M. Sherraden (Baltimore: Johns Hopkins University Press, 2001). Copyright 2001; used by permission.

the roles of the market and the state and to the serious limitations and consequences of promoting productive aging.

The Development of the Productive Aging Perspective

During the 1960s and 1970s, social movements played a significant role in shaping and promoting the public agenda in areas of racial and gender equality. Popular movements for the promotion of health and aging also grew out of the same environment, which fostered a renewed emphasis on individual rights, collective obligation, and state responsibility. However, the 1980s, under the leadership of President Ronald Reagan, were marked by a resurgence of market ideology, individual responsibility, and devolution of the state (Estes, 1991b). These concepts were vigorously promoted by private sector business and institutionalized through laws. Previous chapters in this volume have explored the influence of these concepts on social benefits, health care, and retirement. Over the course of time, these ideological concepts have been incorporated into the promotion of health and aging as well.

Recognizing the Social Determinants of Health

The 1970s marked a watershed in understanding the importance of social, environmental, and behavioral determinants of health status. Dubos (1979), McKeown (1978), and Belloc and Breslow (1972) contributed to an increased understanding of the social determinants of health, particularly the role of environment, social class and other social factors, and lifestyle as major determinants of individual health status. Dubos's pioneering work addressed individual adaptation to the social and physical environment. McKeown demonstrated the role of improved nutrition, changing personal habits, and sanitation in achieving the marked improvements in health status during the past 150 years, calling into question the strong belief that improved medical care and technology have been the major source of health gains. Belloc and Breslow (1972) demonstrated an association between lifestyle habits and physical health status, supporting the promotion of individual behavior change as part of preventive health principles. Physical health was measured in terms of disability, chronic conditions, impairments, symptoms, and energy level. Positive behaviors for health were sleeping 7 or 8 hours each night, maintaining normal weight, engaging in physical exercise, not smoking cigarettes, and moderate alcohol consumption.

McKinlay and McKinlay (1977) added credence to these arguments by showing that at most only 3.5% of the total decline in mortality (for the eight infectious diseases they studied) since 1900 could be ascribed to medical measures. They found, instead, that social factors, including a rise in income and better sanitation and nutrition, were more significant in improving the health of the U.S. population than medical interventions, including both prevention and treatment.

Addressing the Health of Older Persons

During this same period, two reports were released that spoke directly to the health of the aging population. The 1977 report of the President's Council on Physical Fitness and Sports states that older persons (a) believe their need for exercise diminishes and eventually disappears with age; (b) exaggerate the risks involved in regular exercise beyond middle age; (c) overrate the benefits of light, irregular exercise; and (d) underrate their own capabilities and abilities to participate in fitness activities (President's Council on Physical Fitness, 1979). For the first time, the 1979 Surgeon General's Report on Health Promotion and Disease Prevention, titled *Healthy People* (U.S. Department of Health, Education, and Welfare [DHEW], 1979) set specific quantifiable national health status goals for the health of older adults: "by 1990, to reduce the average annual number of days of restricted activity due to chronic and acute conditions by 204 to fewer than thirty days per year for people aged 65 and older" (U.S. DHEW, 1979, p. 71). This document laid out a conceptual framework for national health promotion activities focusing on individual behavior and lifestyle as a major determinant of health and illness.

In 1981, Minkler and Fullarton noted that despite the national promotion of this framework, the elderly were excluded from health promotion programs because these programs focused on (a) life extension, while at the same time the elderly were perceived as not having a future; (b) reducing risk factors associated with premature mortality and morbidity, whereas many of the elderly had already lived beyond risk of premature death; (c) the prevention of signs of aging and the maintenance of youth, making "old folks" unwelcome; and (d) absence and avoidance of chronic disease, which did not speak to the elderly population who already had one or more chronic conditions.

Simultaneously, Fries (1980) observed that the increased incidence of chronic disease occurred because people are more likely to survive illnesses that once led to mortality early in life. Because chronic disease is now the major cause of death, he argued that the major emphasis of health care must shift from the treatment of acute illness toward the removal of risk factors associated with chronic illness (Fries, 1980). Because lifestyle is a major risk factor associated with the onset of chronic illness and the resulting functional disability, Fries postulates that modification of lifestyle and behavior to promote health could alter the process of aging; improve the physical, mental, and social functioning of the elderly; reduce disability normally associated with aging; and extend a vigorous life up to the end of what was described as the natural biological life span.

"Successful Aging" as a New Model for Health Promotion

During the late 1970s and early 1980s, the rising interest in health promotion provided a hopeful sign that public health policy would shift (or at least somewhat rebalance priorities) from the dominant biomedical definition and model of health and disease toward a broader bio-psycho social view that encompassed the social and physical environment, as well as individual lifestyle and behavior (McKeown, 1978). Toward such an aim, the Kaiser Family Foundation supported several major initiatives, including (a) work by Green and colleagues (Green, Kreuter, Deeds, & Partridge, 1980) on a model of health promotion that combined health education with related organizational and politico-economic interventions designed to facilitate behavioral and environmental adaptations to improve or protect health and (b) a project on the links between health and community (Amick, Levine, Tarlov, & Walsh, 1995; Haan, Kaplan, & Syme, 1989). The 1981 White House Conference on Aging (WHCoA) recommended increased governmental, voluntary, and private sector activity in health promotion and fitness for the elderly (WHCoA, 1981).

Advances in gerontological theorizing and research were consistent with the efforts of health promotion advocates to improve individual outcomes as they increased individual choices and personal control. The 1980s saw an energizing of gerontology with the notion of the "plasticity" (even the potential reversibility) of aging, the differentiation of "usual" aging from "successful aging" (Rowe & Kahn, 1987), and the idea of the modifiability of previously considered inevitable biological, behavioral, and social processes. The well-received optimism about aging continues with the MacArthur Foundation Network on Successful Aging (Rowe & Kahn, 1998) and the findings of Manton, Corder, and Stallard (1997) regarding the decline in the prevalence of chronic disability among the elderly.

In the case of successful aging, the new positive framework points to the identification of individual risk factors for unsuccessful aging and to successful health-promoting behavior choices. Prima facie, the work theoretically challenges the biomedical paradigm, while recognizing the importance of social and environmental factors in making successful aging a possibility. Unfortunately, the model of successful aging has several limitations because the social and environmental factors necessary to successfully age remain underexplicated, undertheorized, and underresearched in the work on successful aging, as they have in the work on health promotion more broadly. Riley (1998) describes these shortcomings well:

> Although it elaborates the potentials for individual success, it fails to develop adequately the social structural opportunities necessary for realizing success.... Changes in lives and changes in social structures are fundamentally interdependent. Thus successful aging involves the interplay between lives and the complementary dynamic of structural change. (p. 151)

Thus, although the promotion of successful aging sought to shift the paradigm of old age health, it failed to address fundamental structures that are integral in actualization of successful aging. Further adaptation of this theory reinforced, rather than addressed, these limitations. One such theory is the concept of productive aging, which sought to locate successful aging within a social context of productivity.

From "Successful" to "Productive" Aging

There are multiple definitions of productive aging, although they are generally compatible with one another. Morgan (1988) defines productivity as activities that produce goods and services that otherwise would have to be paid for and that reduce the demand on goods and services produced by others. Herzog and colleagues define productive aging as any activity that produces goods or services, whether paid for or not, including activities such as housework, child care, volunteer work, and help to family and friends (Herzog, Kahn, Morgan, Jackson, & Antonucci, 1989). According to Bass, Caro, and Chen (1993), the focus of productive aging is primarily on social and economic production of goods and services that create value (paid for or not) and on developing the capacity to produce them (paid for or not). With productive aging, it is said that there is (or will be) a sense of achievement and life engagement and a view of older adults as a major and valuable resource. Finally, Butler and Schechter (1995) define productive aging as the capacity for an individual or a population to serve in the paid workforce, to serve in volunteer activities, to assist in the family, and to maintain oneself as independently as possible. The aging are viewed individually and collectively as a resource to meet their own and society's needs.

A Critique

Well-intentioned and developed by leading scholars in the field of gerontology, the concept of productive aging seeks a positive recognition of the resources of old age. The concept is designed by gerontologists to show that old people remain productive, thus seeking to reverse the "decline and loss" paradigm associated with aging. This new construct seeks to counteract the greedy-geezer stereotypes by showing that old people are contributing to society and are not simply selfish consumers (Holstein, 1999). However, these ideas "[affirm] a cultural ideal—that it is good to elevate productivity as a ruling metaphor for a good old age" (Holstein, 1999, p. 359), and as Holstein argues, this is where the problems with productive aging begin.

The theoretical model of social policy and aging helps illuminate the limitations of a productive aging perspective by examining the assumptions and values behind the concept of "productivity" as applied to the aging process. The prioritization of the market and the reliance on the underlying value of individual responsibility are consistent with and reinforced by neoliberal and neoconservative ideologies (see Chapter 5 for a detailed discussion on these perspectives). Likewise, the perspective perpetuates the microlevel interpretation of health and pays inadequate attention to the macrostructural factors. Finally the inter-locking systems of oppression that result in health inequalities are ignored by the model of productive aging (see Chapter 7 for more discussion of these inequalities). Thus, the application of productivity to old age has the potential to negatively affect the elderly (i.e., create new problems) and reduce resource allocations to them by creating a greater sense of individual accountability and responsibility for the costs and conse-quences of unproductive aging.

Promoting the Role of the Market in Addressing Health

Production is a core feature of any market-based analysis (Marx, 1887/1978). Thus, the concept of productive aging is consistent with, if not an extension of, the ideology of the market into the aging process. Directly or indirectly, the productivity movement in aging is entirely consistent with the larger political-economic context in which the market is seen as the best (or only) way to meet social needs. The "giving away" of the public sphere and public responsibility for the aging is thus done at high cost. Defining aging as productive is a capitulation to the power of the market, rendering up all human experience (and liv-ing) to (and subject to) controls of the market and as "work" (perhaps at any price). Productive aging paves the way for the extension of the market mentality (and its purportedly politically neutral "invisible hand" or inexorable laws of competition) into judgments about do-ing housework, caring for others, and, by extension, those personal health behaviors necessary to productively age (i.e., diet, exercise, and not smoking).

Two characteristics of market ideology are central to the critique of the productive aging: individualism and commodification. Under market logic, the individual has complete authority over the produc-tion of goods and services, thus constructing a normative view of aging. The onus for productive aging is on the individual, not on soci-ety or the state. The ideology of individualism is at the heart of the re-surgence of the market, in which preference for the market far out-weighs considerations of the growing inequalities being produced in U.S. society. Because what is valued is what is produced rather than who is producing it, how it is produced, or under what circumstances, what disappears is any notion of value or meaning detached from economic worth and defined according to capitalist logic. Also what disappears is legitimacy for the notion of "social need" or deserving-ness based on human condition or social need. Such a transfer of responsibility is consistent with other efforts to reduce state obligation. The movement to enhance elder productivity, which inevitably confounds successful aging with productivity, provides the necessary cognitive framework for the retreat of the state and for cuts in Medicare and Social Security. In this way, the concept of productive aging may be useful in advancing the interests of those who wish to contain and roll-back the welfare state. Embracing the concept and policy of productive aging risks the obliteration of all other values except the economic metric. This approach threatens to redefine every stage of the life course as being required to meet productivity standards in ways that allow for the imposition of the norms of production.

Limitations of a Microlevel Approach

The application of the productivity notion for what the best of aging "is" may transfer the risk from the state to the individual and from the community to the older person. The rubric of productive aging is predicated on the concept of responsibility at the individual level—consistent with the individualization of risk, apart from all of the social forces and social factors (race, class, and gender) that significantly shape and determine the differential exposure to risk (health risks and other types of risks) and how that risk is individually experienced (as well as with the economic and political weapons to combat it).

The concept of productive aging supports the idea of aging as a problem of individuals. It is subject to interpretations that begin and end on the individual level, with the individual seen (and blamed) as productive or unproductive. The measures of evaluation are at the individual level. Matilda Riley (1998) speaks to this "problem" by stressing the vital importance of thinking and working on societal and institutional levels (e.g., of schools, employers, churches, government) as well as on the individual level.

The use of the productive aging concept obfuscates what is a macro problem—a society that stigmatizes and "throws away" a particular age segment (and more) of its people—and redefines it as a micro problem of individuals who are aging. Holstein (1992) has identified the negative effect of the concept, especially for people who suffer chronic health problems or major disabilities because these outcomes are the result of a failure to "productively age." The most tangible focus remains on the individual to make changes to his or her lifestyle by being energized and motivated to work (paid or unpaid) and to exercise and improve one's nutrition, improve one's stress control, reduce one's use of alcohol and drugs, and quit smoking—independent of real and meaningful changes in the larger structural arrangements.

Perpetuation of the Biomedicalization of Health, the Medical-Industrial Complex, and the Aging Enterprise

The attention to aging at the individual level is consistent with the biomedical perspective discussed in Chapter 3. With the aging of the population, the highly profitable biomedically oriented, medical-industrial complex (Estes, Harrington, & Davis, 1992) and aging enterprise remain intact and unchallenged (see Chapter 8 for more discussion). Insofar as health promotion and lifestyle behaviors converge or are defined synonymously with (or antecedent to) productive aging, a vast new array of private sector product lines and industries to promote dietary, exercise, and other behavioral changes—primarily aimed at the individual level—are legitimated by the aging enterprise. The economic and social resources to avail oneself of these are likely to continue to be determined on the basis of the market or the ability to pay for them privately rather than as a right to health or well-being in old age. The profits of the corporate enterprise eclipse the state resources that might be applied to ensure economic security in old age.

Thus, although the concepts of productive aging have been successful in promoting the preeminence of market-based solutions and individual responsibility, they have done little to change the actual provision of health care services. Despite the accumulating research evidence documenting the import of social as opposed to medical factors in health and aging, as well as fledgling health promotion efforts, the hegemony of the medical model in health and aging policy in the United States persists. Major health care policies for the aging continue to reflect the biomedical definition of health in which health is seen as the absence of disease, whereas disease is seen as a deviation from a biological norm of a young and "healthy" society and aging is seen as a biologically determined process of inevitable decline. Health maintenance is thus focused on treating these processes of disease and decline. More recently, a perceptible yet subtle shift has been to treating the "risk factors" for these processes of disease and decline.

With the "biomedicalization of aging" (Estes & Binney, 1989), old age is constructed as a disease and aging is portrayed as a medical problem requiring more and more medical services. This biomedicalization has contributed to the acute care bias of Medicare and the failure of health policy to provide long-term care and the rehabilitative and social supportive services needed by the chronically ill. More important, it diverts resources and attention from other factors that have a greater influence on determining the experience and quality of life of older persons—an adequate income and a safe and secure physical environment, among others. And finally, the biomedicalization of aging has contributed substantially to the expansion of multiple highly profitable medical industries and professions that provide acute and high-tech care to the elderly—the aging enterprise and the medical-industrial complex (Estes, 1979).

To sum up, although knowledge of the determinants of health in the aging process has grown and health promotion and disease prevention programs have also grown in visibility in Congress, in federal agencies, and at state and local levels of government, policies that build on this knowledge and perspective remain frustratingly illusive to the American people. The surgeon general's recent report, *Healthy People 2010* (U.S. Department of Health and Human Services [DHHS], 1998), and recent Medicare legislation (the 1997 Balanced Budget Act) contain new coverage of a number of preventive benefits (e.g., the full cost of mammograms, prostate cancer screening). These efforts have been aided by many groups outside government, including the Institute of Medicine of the National Academy of Sciences and a growing number of university and business interests. Private sector groups actively advocating for health promotion include voluntary professional health organizations, health and life insurance companies, fitness and health food industries, and some employers. Nevertheless, health policy that actually promotes health (rather than being bounded by a sickness model) receives limited support or funding, in large part because of the difficulty of cracking the already medically controlled and potentially volatile financing of the big categorical health programs such as Medicare and Medicaid. Current policy thus represents a formidable obstacle to the advancement of health and aging policy that would truly challenge the medical model with health goals that would maximize the likelihood of successful or productive aging.

Perpetuation of Inequalities From the Systems of Oppression

Previous chapters of this volume have demonstrated that economic status, race/ethnicity, and gender profoundly affect an older adult's ability to experience a meaningful and productive aging experience. Dramatically reduced incomes, decreased power and social standing, the threat of economic and social dependency, chronic illness, the loss of social support systems, and the loss of control over individual life-style are all powerful determinants of the well-being of the elderly in our society. Researchers have repeatedly demonstrated the importance of social class (socioeconomic status) in every measure of health at every stage of life and aging (House, Kessler, & Herzog, 1990). However, as discussed in length in Chapters 6 and 7, race/ethnicity and gender also play important roles in the calculation. Thus, structural elements such as class, race, and gender are central in shaping whatever may be possible in "productively" aging.

Productive aging cannot be separated from the larger issues of society's policy development and choices across income, housing, and other social issues in regard to aging: the social, economic, and political environment in which individuals age. There is a link between success-ful and productive aging in the sense that people who are successfully aging can be productive and contribute to our society. There are formi-dable social, structural, and institutional impediments to "making it" as a productive "ager." The concept of productive aging tends to ignore gender and race/ethnicity inequalities and different life chances. It also glosses over the opportunities afforded (or not) under these different circumstances and the explicit social policies that create, for example, high rates of poverty for older women in the United States and even higher poverty levels for women of color.

The linking or confounding of positive aging with productivity is likely to have unintended but discriminatory effects against older people as well as others who live outside a well-defined normative mainstream, particularly those on the margins; those who are "not normal," perhaps disabled; the oldest old; and those without resources, especially minorities, the poor, and women. Holstein (1992) argues, persuasively, that the focus on productive aging will truncate rather than expand an older woman's chance to construct a meaningful last chapter of her life. Furthermore, she argues, the definition perpetuates a perception of perceived personal and social needs that is especially damaging to women.

Constructions of Reality

Labels or social constructions of reality are crucial in defining "the problem" and the policy solutions attendant to the problem. The importance of labels applied to the elderly has been well documented (Estes, 1979). There are competing constructions of reality regarding what is productive or successful aging. The consequences of these competing definitions, labels, and constructions have to be considered. Moody (1988a, 1993a) has alluded to the inescapable semantic significance of the phrase "productive aging" and the problem of there being narrow standards for defining a productive life.

Paradoxically, through the concept of productive aging, a negative concept of people who are failures may be socially adopted. This is so because the concept implicitly accords normative value to aging equated with success. Lack of productive aging equals failure—failure to produce goods or services, whether paid or unpaid—and potentially the obligation to produce more, particularly more of the "free" labor of elder caregiving that women already provide in large quantities (Estes & Binney, 1989). The concept of "productive aging" lulls society into believing that there are no losers—that productive aging is a positive goal synonymous with apple pie and motherhood (Estes & Binney, 1989). The productivity label (being so or not so) is likely to contribute to the already worrisome construction of aging as a burden. It is consonant with the constructions of aging as a demographic and fiscal crisis—as a burden that the nation (i.e., especially the government) cannot bear.

Conclusion

In a capitalist society where the market is primary and value is what is monetized (in terms of dollars produced), there are risks and formidable political, economic, and social barriers to the proposed reevaluation of what elders "do" under the productive aging banner. Whether intentional or not, the concept of productive aging promotes the role of the market in addressing health-reinforcing, individual-based solutions and obfuscating the role of the state in addressing the structures that limit individuals' ability to actualize aging. This market-based approach also perpetuates the biomedicalization of health and strengthens the role of the medical-industrial complex and the aging enterprise. Finally, as a result, the perpetuation of inequalities associated with race/ethnicity, class, and gender and the promotion of negative social constructions of aging are perpetuated.

Although the idea of "productive aging" speaks broadly to the social, environmental, behavioral, and other factors involved, it underplays the profoundly difficult task of truly conceptualizing what it would take in the form of altered policy and social/economic arrangements (and redistribution) to achieve the measure of their promise. It is unclear how productive aging will achieve environmental or policy changes needed to support healthy aging lifestyles because on the policy level, the concept of productive aging does little to challenge the status quo. There are no accompanying or requisite economic or health policies to address problems of market failure or of unequal access to whatever is defined as "productive aging."

In contrast, however, if the field of aging is to truly promote productive aging, there is a need for enlarged public and private sector responsibility. Community and social institutional responsibility (including policy changes and resource commitments) are essential elements of any program to promote productive aging in order to permit and promote positive individual and societal outcomes. Otherwise, the certain outcome will be the continuous reproduction of inequalities of race, class, and gender, with the increased exacerbation of the losses incurred in old age.

10 The Underdevelopment of Community-Based Services in the U.S. Long-Term Care System

A Structural Analysis

Marty Lynch
Carroll L. Estes

The aging of the population and the growing number of younger disabled persons ensure a growing demand for health and long-term care services as described in Chapter 7. Although the disabled consistently express a clear preference to remain in their own homes, eschewing nursing home institutionalization, community-based and home-delivered long-term care services are relatively underdeveloped. Currently, over 70% of government expenditures for long-term care services are spent on nursing home care; thus, publicly financed resources are devoted predominantly to institutional care (Braden et al., 1998).

This chapter locates the underdevelopment of community-based long-term care within a larger political and economic context, predicated on the assumptions that such services do not develop in a vacuum and that the policies shaping these services develop within a broader structural reality. Economic, political, and sociocultural factors have influenced the development of long-term care systems in the United

States and to a great extent delineated future directions of policy and service delivery development.

Aging and Disability in the United States

In 1990, 13% of the U.S. population was aged 65 or older. Of the growing older population, those 85 years of age and older (the oldest old) are most likely to need long-term care services, both institutional and community based. The number and proportion of the oldest old has grown most rapidly. In 1994, 3 million Americans were aged 85 or older and represented nearly 10% of the elderly population (U.S. Bureau of the Census, 1996). According to the Census Bureau's "middle series" projections, those aged 85 and over will more than quadruple between 2000 and 2050, to 19 million, composing 24% of the elderly (U.S. Bureau of the Census, 2000). The impact of these figures on the growth of the long-term care industry may be understood by looking at the rates of elders with disabilities. In 1991, estimates are that 17% (5.3 million) of noninstitutionalized elders aged 65 and older required some assistance with either activities of daily living (ADLs) or instrumental activities of daily living (IADLs). Approximately 14% of elders aged 65 to 74 have some level of disability compared with 58.2% of those over the age of 85. Only 2.7% of those aged 65 to 84 are institutionalized in a nursing home, whereas 18% of the oldest old (aged 85+) are (American Association of Retired Persons [AARP], 1994). Less than 1% of elders resided in board-and-care homes (Sirrocco, 1994).

Long-term care expenditures for nursing home care were $83 billion in 1997 (Braden et al., 1998), and it is projected that these will grow to $98 billion by the year 2020 (Rivlin & Wiener, 1988). Current expenditures for home care services are $8.6 billion, and these figures are expected to grow to $21.9 billion by 2020. Home care services may include supportive social services, respite care, and adult day health care, but it is difficult to obtain expenditure data on the full array of community-based long-term care programs now developing. Community-based care, other than that delivered by home health agencies and in-home support service programs, makes up a very small proportion of overall long-term care expenditures in the United States.

Projections of the graying of the United States are underscored by recent data on the continuing decline of mortality. On the basis of the government's Long Term Care Survey, Manton, Singer, and Suzman (1993) report the finding that mortality declines for persons 85 years of age and older, just between 1988 and 1991 alone, are in excess of 8.6%. Projections for an older population exceeding 20% of the population by 2020 (as noted in Chapter 7) have been accompanied by a debate concerning whether the observed mortality declines are positive or negative, the answer to which turns on whether there are commensurate changes (decline or delay) in disability prevalence and whether there is a compression of morbidity. Nevertheless, under all scenarios, there will be absolute increases in the need for long-term care because even the most optimistic projections of disability declines in future cohorts of aging "do not wholly compensate for population aging" (Manton, Singer & Suzman, 1993). In addition, significant high-risk subgroups among the elderly are not going to diminish, particularly the lower socioeconomic classes, minorities, and women. To the extent that there are increases in the number of disabled elderly who wish to reside in the community, there will be a need for changes in the mix of long-term care services—notably, an increasing demand for community-based care (e.g., in-home and adult day care) and equipment use (Manton, Corder, & Stallard, 1993).

The extension of life expectancy has created a number of new problems (LaPlante, 1991), such as chronic illness and the thinning of social supports that are not particularly amenable to solution by the present policy-driven acute medical model of health care. It is necessary to design and test models of long-term care that differ fundamentally from the acute care model that dominates health policy, particularly in view of the fact that dependency may be either increased or decreased by policy interventions and their consequences.

In the 21st century with its demographic changes, issues of individual and population dependency are paramount. The fear that the growing older population will place catastrophic burdens on society and deplete health care resources has been termed "apocalyptic demography" (Robertson, 1999). This fear and the shape of the long-term care system designed to meet the needs of elders are deeply influenced by the political economy of the society.

Rowe and Kahn (1987) make an important distinction between extrinsic aging that is modifiable (environmentally, behaviorally, and socially induced aging) and intrinsic aging (inherent genetic/biological processes). As described in Chapter 7, dependency in old age is not a "given" but is a product of both intrinsic and extrinsic aging. An unknown degree of dependency in old age is extrinsic and is modifiable, preventable, or reversible (Rowe & Kahn, 1987; see also Chapter 9). Social policy is an example of a major extrinsic factor that affects dependency in old age.

Long-Term Care and Community-Based Care

The long-term care system that currently exists in the United States can be analyzed from a number of perspectives. Some key perspectives are suggested by analysis of the health care system (McKinlay, 1985). This framework is equally applicable to long-term care. Building on this work and the theoretical model presented in Chapter 1, long-term care is viewed from the following perspectives:

1. The financial and industrial capital, including corporations and the individuals and interests controlling them
2. The state in capitalist society as it ensures accumulation of private economic gain, deals with preserving social harmony (maintaining legitimacy of the state), promotes the dominance of a market ideology, and produces legislation that furthers these ends
3. The level of the delivery system for health and long-term care services, including the professionals and organizations involved in service delivery
4. The public, including users of long-term care, their family members who are involved in providing most of the nation's long-term care, and other members of the society who may one day find themselves in the position of either user or caregiver

Financial and Industrial Capital

Long-term care services are of interest to large corporate and business interests at several levels. These include the societal cost of reproducing the workforce, worker productivity issues, worker benefits, issues of maintaining cordial but dominant relations with employees, and opportunities for profit making (see also Chapter 8).

First is the cost of reproducing the workforce. In some manner, business and the society as a whole must provide the necessary conditions to continue to produce an available workforce. For the most part, long-term care services are required by older persons who are no longer in the paid labor force. However, care for the elderly can be seen as part of a broader socially defined range of conditions needed to maintain the working population. In addition, a significant number of younger disabled people in the society may either be seen as dependent or, in some cases, may be employed as productive workers. These younger disabled people (estimated to make up more than 40% of the population in need of long-term care) also require a range of long-term care services. Business itself has traditionally taken little responsibility for older workers who are disabled. Although some businesses have paid for health care benefits for employees and retirees, the proportion of firms providing these benefits are shrinking, and for the most part, they do not cover long-term care services. Only 7% of the cost of long-term care was paid by private insurance in 1997 (Braden et al., 1998), and there is no estimate on the part of the 7% paid by employers. It is likely to be insignificant.

Corporate America has also had an interest in promoting legislated retirement policies (Walker, 1984) so that older, less productive workers could be removed from the workforce in times of high unemployment and competition for profits. The costs of workers can be reduced by downsizing and the casualization of labor, increasing the percentage of temporary and part-time workers without benefits. With labor market flexibility, employers may open up positions for younger and presumably more productive (and lower-cost) employees. The welfare state has developed the Social Security system to provide financial incentives and justification for this transition out of the economically productive workforce and into retirement.

Some corporations, such as IBM and AMEX, have begun to develop benefit programs related to long-term care services. Two common approaches have been the promotion of private long-term care insurance to be purchased by today's workers for their future needs and the provision of programs to assist employees with care of older dependents. Employee assistance programs, when they are available, provide professional assistance to employees in finding long-term care resources. They are aimed at reducing absenteeism and the stress related to dependent care and thus improving productivity of the workforce. They may also be part of an overall benefit package necessary to attract and maintain a highly skilled workforce.

Efforts to encourage employees to purchase long-term care coverage for themselves are consistent with the U.S. market ideology of individuals' taking financial responsibility for their own health and long-term care needs while bolstering a profitable private insurance industry. The growth of private insurance solutions would have the positive benefit for corporations of reducing pressures for a publicly financed system of long-term care (as a right or entitlement) in ways that might drain more of corporate profits into taxes.

Although a small number of firms offer long-term care benefits, most corporate interests have resisted taking any direct responsibility for long-term care costs. Corporations have allowed the state to take responsibility for the poorest of those needing long-term care through the Medicaid program and to shunt the remaining burden to the individuals and families involved as their own private responsibility. Near-poor elders in need of long-term care, particularly those most exploited during their working years, women and minorities, and those living alone are often left to fend for themselves.

Corporate interests in U.S. society have a major stake in how long-term care services are delivered. According to this perspective, long-term care should be delivered in such a way that it does not question the dominant market ideology of U.S. society. From the political economy perspective, long-term care provision is consistent with existing structural realities. It is partially state supported but reinforces an ideology consistent with a market approach. What does this mean? Long-term care is delivered in a way that supports opportunities for profits to be made from its delivery; it involves finance capital through the insurance, pharmaceutical, and other industries; it reinforces the concept of private versus public responsibility; and it involves an important role for the profession of medicine as a trusted partner (Ehrenreich & Ehrenreich, 1978; Parsons, 1951).

Long-term care becomes a more important opportunity for corporate investment as the number of disabled elders grows. Elderly needs affect worker productivity, worker demands, and the potential claims on the state for provision of services (which, if not addressed, may cause the state to encounter its own legitimacy problems). Long-term care has the potential to both place a greater demand on the corporate sector and allow for financial gain for a relatively small part of that sector.

The Role of the State

As described in Chapter 1, O'Connor (1973), Habermas (1973), and others discuss two principal functions of the state in late capitalist society:

1. The *accumulation* function, whereby the state must ensure the continued profitable working of the capitalist economy
2. The *legitimation* function, requiring the state to maintain its own legitimacy by responding to the needs of its citizens.

O'Connor suggests that in the age of monopoly capital, ever-expanding state expenditures on social capital, or developing societal infrastructure, are required to increase or maintain profitability for corporate America. At the same time, increasing the number of workers who do not share in the profits and accumulated wealth of the corporate sector requires state-provided benefits and services. In times of economic crisis and global competition, increased state funds are required simultaneously for both profitable accumulation and for additional funding to support the welfare functions of the state. A greater number of workers are squeezed out of the economy at the same time as there is financial pressure on the state budgets (at every governmental level: federal, state, and local) to contract spending on welfare and social assistance (legitimation) functions. By the late 1990s, the U.S. economy was booming and there was a significant decline in unemployment, but many of the millions of new jobs are low paying, without benefits or career opportunities. Yet demands for fiscal discipline have continued in federal efforts to balance the budget and reduce Medicare and Medicaid spending (Lynch & Minkler, 1999). These reductions have created continued pressure on the welfare and service functions of the state at the same time as corporate wealth as measured by stock values has increased dramatically.

According to O'Connor (1973), the state budgeting process is an important arena for class and other social struggles in times of economic crisis and constraint (which may be generated by economic or political forces). This is particularly so when resources are, on the one hand, limited and, on the other hand, needed or demanded by capital and the corporate sector to support accumulation functions. At such times, social spending comes under heavy attack by corporate and politically conservative interests. The social contract between big business, big labor, and government, present in economic boom times, breaks down as the economy tightens. Given the enormous wealth accumulation and growing inequality of the late 1990s and accompanying attacks on welfare, Social Security, and other government programs, it is clear that such attacks are not limited to times of economic crisis alone. The distribution and exercise of political power is highly influential in setting the course of events.

The role of the state in the underdevelopment of community-based long-term care systems can be analyzed in light of its broader, generic responsibilities. Expansion of long-term care services for disabled elders plays a minimal (though growing) role in the accumulation process. Long-term care services could be seen as part of the necessary cost of society's infrastructure to reproduce the capitalist economy and maintain the legitimacy of the state. The necessity for long-term care to the accumulation process is much less direct than the education of future workers or the provision of health and social services to children and younger adults so they can become productive or maintain their productivity. Up to the present, long-term care services for the most part are a social expense required to maintain the legitimacy of the state.

The development (and underdevelopment) of state welfare programs is not totally driven by economic considerations but also depends greatly on the strength and organization of working people in the society (Navarro & Berman, 1983). Pressure for long-term care reform, including improvement and coverage of community-based services, comes from progressive organizations attempting an expansion of the legitimation function. Despite the demographic imperative discussed earlier and mounting pressure from advocates (Families USA, Gray Panthers, AARP), chances of any major expansion of long-term care coverage at the federal government level are slim at this time (Estes, Wiener, Goldberg, & Goldensen, 2000) because of the discouraging failure of Clinton's health reform effort in 1993-1994, the conservatism of Congress, the ratcheting down of welfare expenditures, and the relatively weak organization of advocacy, labor, and political groups in the United States. On the other hand, corporate and other dominant political interests argue that long-term care coverage would be too costly and would displace the appropriate care of family members and other informal caregivers, usually women. Economists call this the "woodwork effect," in which people give up the caregiving work they are doing and demand that it be provided by the formal service providers. The stalemate over long-term care policy means that current costs are born heavily by those providing care at home and are not faced directly either by business or by the state.

The struggle to develop support for community-based long-term care faces not only economic class issues (because those who are well-off are more likely to be able to pay for care) but also major gender and racial equity issues because policymakers tend to be affluent white men who are less concerned about burdens typically borne by women and low-income or minority elders. Also important is the issue that, outside the formal home health agency sector and some retirement communities, for-profit corporate providers continue to have a limited role in developing community-based models of care. This type of long-term care is thus not yet a major opportunity for profitable accumulation. By contrast, for-profits own 67% of all nursing homes (Harrington, 1999) and maintain a powerful lobbying force to protect their business interests through influencing state regulation and reimbursement policies.

Efforts to expand governmental support for long-term care funding have been faced with generalized attacks on the welfare state made during the Carter, Reagan, and Bush presidencies (Navarro, 1984). The pressures against expansion of government programs continued throughout Clinton's presidency. The welfare state and social spending have been blamed by conservative politicians for budget deficits and the supposed economic crisis of the overall economic system (Marmor, Mashaw, & Harvey, 1990). Attacks on the welfare expenditures have come not only in the form of reduction of funds but in efforts to privatize and corporatize service expenditures and heavily promote a market ideology in the delivery of services (Estes, Binney, & Bergthold, 1989b). Navarro describes this process not as a dismantling of the welfare state but as a restructuring process. As state expenditures for social services are reduced, funds are shifted to military or criminal justice programs, and funds that remain available are shifted from public to private provision of services. Additional changes are made within government in terms of how funds are managed and allocation decisions made. Navarro (1984) states that this restructuring of the welfare state is backed up by a capitalist ideological offensive. The ideological process includes an attempt to lower people's expectations, focus on individual lifestyles, blame the victims of social problems, and promote self-care.

In long-term care, these attacks are paralleled (a) by efforts to suggest that family (i.e., women) rather than government or business should be the responsible party for providing long-term care and that it is the individual's responsibility to provide for such needs by opening individual retirement accounts (IRAs), buying private long-term care insurance, and the like and (b) by intimating that older people who require long-term care assistance somehow failed by not providing adequate resources for their own care. All of these attacks deflect attention away from the state's social responsibilities and from capital's failure to pay the cost for the reproduction of the labor force.

In the 1990s, the Clinton administration twice proposed long-term care coverage reforms, once for community-based long-term care support as part of broader health reform efforts (Estes, Wiener, Goldberg, & Goldensen, 2000) and, second, for much more modest caregiver support through tax credits and support programs. In both instances, these reform proposals have been paired with efforts to support the expansion of private long-term care insurance either through tax credits, education, or federal employee benefit programs. Despite the fact that both efforts involved support for private, insurance-based solutions (a little for private insurance in the case of a Clinton health reform community-based service proposal, which was largely publicly funded, and a lot for private insurance in the 1999 effort), neither reform succeeded. Failure of reform efforts at the federal level has been accompanied by devolution of responsibility to the state level, and most of all the continuing and growing pressure on those who provide unpaid informal care (see also Chapters 6 and 11). Several progressive states (Oregon, Minnesota, New York, Massachusetts, and others) have attempted to shift the balance of long-term care services to the community-based arena by developing new service options and care coordination efforts for their Medicaid populations (Coleman, 1998; Mollica & Riley, 1997). These reforms have been accomplished under the rubric of achieving costs savings while responding to consumer demands. In some states, they have accompanied moves to privatize Medicaid service delivery by turning over program responsibilities to managed care companies. Growing interest in managed long-term care parallels managed care growth for employer-sponsored health care benefits, behavioral or mental health care, Medicare, and Medicaid for nondisabled populations.

Professionals and Delivery Systems in Long-Term Care

The sociology of health care has traditionally paid great attention to the role of the physician and physician dominance in health care (Freidson, 1970, 1989; McKinlay, 1985; Parsons, 1951). Long-term care as it is currently configured is deeply influenced by the power of the medical profession to define and "treat" the condition of aging (Estes & Binney, 1989). Skilled nursing facilities rely on the involvement (fleeting though it may be) of physicians to certify illness and legitimate care plans, ensure quality, and provide at least minimal clinical care for patients. This symbolic presence ensures medical social control. In addition, physicians are often intimately involved in the decision to institutionalize patients. At a structural level, some nursing homes are privately owned on a for-profit basis by physicians. At the level of home care agencies, physicians provide the orders that allow for reimbursement under medically dominated insurance programs such as Medicare and most private insurance.

Despite strong legal and regulatory involvement in long-term care, physicians have traditionally been less interested in treating long-term chronic health problems of older people. Western medicine relies on a dominant ideology of positivist science. That ideology sees the physician as a scientist who diagnoses specific acute problems, resolves or treats them, and moves on. In addition, the physician in Parsons's (1951) view has a role in legitimating the sick role and returning the patient to productive functioning. The very chronic debilitating nature of the problems facing those elders in need of long-term care service negates this role for the physician. The physician is not going to be able to cure the problem; the patient's functional problems are, for the most part, visually obvious, requiring only physician certification for reimbursement purposes; and there is little opportunity for the patient's return to productive functioning in the economic sphere.

Chronic health problems, according to Strauss and Corbin (1988), involve much more than a single acute episode. The process of chronic illness and disability is long-term and requires management and coordination of services by a broad range of parties. The patient, the family, informal caregivers, poorly paid attendants, and social service workers become much more important than the physician except in acute episodes of the problem. The physician, despite controlling the legitimation of illness and access to many of the available financial resources (reimbursement), is only one member of a larger team. Delivery of community-based long-term care raises these contradictions to a heightened level. State laws and bureaucrats who enforce health law give legitimating power to the physician. Corporate long-term care institutional providers, both for-profit and nonprofit, work with the physician as employee and sometimes partner in their facilities and home health enterprises. For-profits have often solicited the necessary involvement of physicians who, for their part, have enthusiastically accepted the opportunity to improve their income. Expansion of community-based long-term care will require involvement of more than physicians; indeed, it will require multiple parties, including social workers, attendants, and family members who are not historically intertwined with the interests of capital and who do not have a favored or legally regulated position of authority and power. These other caregivers are not either key employees or trusted partners in the accumulation process of business.

Both the more delimited physician's role in the delivery of community-based long-term care and the potential broadening of the authorizing and control mechanisms to other formal and informal care providers make insurance companies, government, and professional medicine wary. Insurance companies fear "moral hazard" where users and family members may ask for formal reimbursed services that they now provide themselves (despite research indicating the reluctance of family caregivers to do this) (Newcomer, Yordi, DuNah, Fox, & Wilkinson, 1999). Government wants to limit expenditures and respond to its major business clients. Medicine does not want a major health-related area such as long-term care to slip from its widening professional hegemony (Relman, 1986).

Once again, a variety of factors within the current professional and long-term care delivery world militate against the major development of community-based long-term care. Community-based care is a sector dominated by professions such as social work and nursing, as well as by advocacy organizations. Models of integrated long-term care are only now developing that allow for profit-making opportunities or for control by the medical profession. Reimbursement policy and provisions, on the other hand, continue to follow an acute biomedical model of care and do not allow payment for the social, coordinative, advocacy, and in-home functions required for long-term chronically ill patients (Wood & Estes, 1988). The medical profession, business, and government are each more comfortable with a skilled nursing institutional model of long-term care that serves as an extension of acute care medicine, allows for ready profit making, and limits social expenditures refereed by the state.

An added factor is the shift during the 1990s toward managed care or health maintenance organization (HMO) models of delivering and financing medical care. HMOs are for the most part large for-profit insurers that have had difficulty providing appropriate care to elders with chronic illness problems and disabilities while reaping considerable profits from the Medicare program (Brown, Clement, Hill, Retchin, & Bergeron, 1993; Lynch & Estes, 1997). It has been suggested that HMO provision of services for the elderly may serve as the velvet glove of rationing (Lynch & Estes, 1997). In addition, the managed care industry has shifted the locus of medical control toward privately traded medical corporations, provoking a backlash from the medical profession and cries for legislation and regulation to protect patients from health care driven by the bottom line. Investor-driven community-based long-term care businesses may raise similar concerns in the future if for-profit institutional long-term care providers broaden their expansion into community service provision.

Conclusion: The Public, Users, and Family Members

Older people and younger advocates for the disabled have stated a clear preference for independent community living even when serious levels of disability exist. The current long-term care system in the United States makes it extremely difficult to respond to this preference. With the great majority of long-term care spending going to institutional nursing home settings and the bulk of home care spending to home health providers, few resources in the current system are left over to support independent living in the community. Medicaid home and community-based waiver service dollars are spent on in-home support services, adult day health care programs, respite, and case management programs offered in some states. These Medicaid services may be provided to poor elders, although many elders, even those below the poverty level, do not receive Medicaid.

Funds provided by the Older Americans Act support another small amount of community-based long-term care services. Few

community-based services are available in general, but they are particularly scarce for near poor elders who cannot afford to pay for adequate
services and do not qualify for Medicaid. Although only 12.5% of
elders fall below the official poverty income level, over 40% fall below
200% of poverty. Women (particularly those widowed and divorced),
minorities, and persons living alone are particularly vulnerable economically (Estes & Michel, 1999).

Individual users of long-term care and their family members face a
bewildering and fragmented array of health, social service, and financial
entitlement programs. They may easily go through several different
assessment, eligibility, and fee-charging processes to obtain needed
services. Very few know much about the available resources or how to
wend their way through the existing bureaucratic maze. The individual
often faces this fragmented system of care at the very time of crisis—
after a hospitalization or after other support has broken down, when he
or she is least able to comprehend or deal with it. Often, the only known
choice of service will be the nursing home, a choice feared by almost all.

Of course, the individual user's chances in the existing long-term
care system have a great deal to do with his or her class standing and
history. Women and minorities, who for the most part are the most
exploited members of our society as workers, become the poorest older
people (see Chapters 6 and 7). They have the fewest resources to buy
services or help to get through the complexities of the system. Because
of their employment history, these groups often rely totally on Social
Security payments and do not have private pensions or significant
savings or investments (Estes & Michel, 1999). In some cases, they have
also held more dangerous and demanding jobs, which have caused
them to have more disabilities and chronic health problems than the
population in general. Those elders who have had more opportunities
during their working life tend to have additional resources and can buy
additional assistance or insurance. Although they must deal with a very
inadequate and fragmented care system, they do so from a more favorable position.

Individuals suffer from a constant ideological bombardment about
the appropriate way to take care of health and long-term care problems.
These messages promote individual responsibility and market-based
approaches that deflect attention away from issues of structural change
in long-term care policy. Despite the dominant ideology, members of
the public in a variety of polls have indicated their willingness to pay

for improved long-term care coverage (Hart & associates, 1990). Many advocacy groups work regularly on this issue, but the progressive movement in the United States has not been strong enough to overcome dominant corporate interests to change long-term care policy.

A universal long-term care system, integrated with a national health program, based in the community, and responding to the interests of users and their families provides a hopeful and contrasting vision to the existing profit and institutionally dominated system (Harrington, Cassel, Estes, Woolhandler, & Himmelstein, 1991). Such a system of long-term care would not alter the basic structural realities of capitalism but would constitute an important victory for working people in the ongoing struggle to improve services and control a greater portion of the state expenditures.

11 The Political Economy of Health Work

Liz Close
Carroll L. Estes
Karen W. Linkins

Systemic characteristics of labor directly involved in the provision of health, social, and long-term care services to older persons in the United States have been repeatedly neglected in policy debates and literature discussions about home health care. Viewing the home as a venue in which acute and chronic elder care is increasingly being provided, this chapter takes a political economy approach to the examination of structural assumptions and arrangements fueling the increasing reliance on informal health workers for the labor inputs ("health work") implicit in the social policy and aging contract for home care.

Sociopolitical assumptions about health work and requisite labor resources have mediated a structural shift of responsibility for health care and social services provision from formal (institutions) to informal (home and community) settings. Workforce and worksite informalization have been well established as an unintended and unanticipated consequence of the Medicare restructuring of reimbursement in the 1980s (Estes, Swan, & associates, 1993). The structural mechanism by which health work (labor) informalization occurred and subsequently has been maintained, however, has not been thoroughly explicated.

Currently, "informal" caregivers routinely perform assessments, procedures, and evaluations in the home for which they generally are neither formally educated nor trained. The primary structural purpose of informal home care is to maintain the elder family member or friend in the home and avoid costly institutionalization. This chapter poses theoretical and practical questions regarding the largely uncontested intersection of paid and unpaid caregivers involved in home health work. The discussion includes a brief theoretical overview of relevant capitalist labor economics, health work cost management, health work informalization, the policy environment, and a beginning explication of the structural interface between formal and informal home health work.

Health Work in the Capitalist Economy

The main topic of this chapter is health work in the form of the labor necessary to provide health, social, and long-term care services to older persons in the home under the auspices of "home health care." Economic concepts germane to this discussion include labor power as a commodity, the relationship of surplus value and profit, productive and unproductive labor, labor supply and demand, and least-cost combinations of workers.

Because labor power itself is a commodity that is bought and sold on the market, its value is determined like that of any other commodity, by the labor time socially necessary for its production (Giddens, 1990). In a capitalist economy, labor power is purchased as a commodity much like any other commodity. A distinct difference is the unit of measurement—the commodity labor power is measured in time, whereas other commodities are measured in tangible units such as weight, volume, or size (Marx, 1887/1978). Importantly, the commodity labor power is also unique because it is, in fact, inseparable from its possessor (the worker).

The rate of surplus value, or rate of exploitation, depends on a baseline of the sociocultural expectations regarding the standards of living in a society. Giddens (1990) maintains that in so presenting profit, Marx unveiled a disguised affiliation—that is, the definite relationship of surplus value and profit. The quest for appropriation of surplus value is a structural source of worker exploitation in capitalist society.

> It motivates the capitalist to keep wages down, to change the work process (by automation and new technologies, close supervision, lengthened work day or overtime, speedups, and dangerous working conditions), and to resist workers' organized attempts to gain higher wages or more control in the workplace. (Waitzkin, 1989, p. 166)

Using Braverman's (1974) conceptualization of the blurring of productive (waged) and unproductive (unwaged) labor, we assume that the "body of workers" engaged in health work for the elderly population necessarily includes productive (paid/formal) and unproductive (unpaid/informal) providers. By doing so, we are able to examine the manner in which the social form of labor—the human labor required for the process of health work production—represents a fashioned and marketable commodity. Marx (1887/1978) noted that the use of the word services instead of wage labor excludes the distinctive characteristic of wage labor and of its use—specifically, that it increases the value of commodities against which it is exchanged; that is, it creates surplus value.

A key point is that by falsely representing services as something other than wage labor, the precise relationship through which money and commodities are transformed into capital is obscured and disregarded. To avoid this pitfall, we consider health work to be provided by wage laborers. Although, by definition, informal caregivers do not receive a wage for the labor power they supply providing health care services, they, nonetheless, possess the capacity to labor for wages, and this necessarily means that their labor has value. Furthermore, and more directly and specifically, the availability of this unpaid labor contributes to the profit margins of hospitals under current Medicare reimbursement schemes in which these facilities "profit" from shorter lengths of stay under the diagnosis-related grouping (DRG) payment policy (also known as the Medicare prospective payment system [PPS]).

Labor economic theory of supply and demand posits that, if there is increased demand for labor power, wages for workers should increase, and, in a competitive market, wage earners should shift to the relatively higher-paying jobs, *ceteris paribus*. A review of literature on wages and benefits in the home care services sector does not indicate that this response occurred even though there has been a rapidly mounting demand placed on the home care labor market with the shift of care from institutions to community-based settings in the post-PPS period (Burbridge, 1993). This incongruity might be explained by the possibility that institutions could have prevented an exodus of personnel by slightly increasing wages and benefits to outpace those offered by community-based agencies. The supply and demand discrepancy might also be due to the availability of informal caregivers to "staff" home care and perform tasks routinely performed by paid personnel inside an institution (bathing, toileting, cooking, feeding, transporting, housecleaning, and administering medical treatments and medications). It is the latter possibility that brings us to the economic principle of "least-cost combination" of labor inputs.

The importance of least-cost combinations (also euphemistically termed "occupational skill mix" in health care circles) to the health worker labor market relates to the economic efficiencies attainable by the optimal combination of human labor inputs to achieve a specific level of output (Feldstein, 1993). In this instance, we assume the level of output to be health, social, and long-term care services necessary to maintain the older client outside of the institutional setting. Szasz (1990) noted that the strategy of varying occupational skill mix in the home care industry to effectively lower personnel costs was impeded by federal reimbursement regulations associated with Medicare policy. This important observation about the formal health care labor sector, however, does not exclude the potential for alterations of skill mix across the formal/informal labor boundary—that is, the shift of necessary labor time between formal and informal providers.

If avenues for decreasing an organization's constant capital outlay are exhausted, the only path open to maintain profit in a capitalist economy is to influence variable capital (the cost of labor power). Assumptions about influencing the cost of labor power by altering occupational skill mix have led to conclusions about the limitations of regulatory controls over to whom and under what conditions reimbursement for services is made (Szasz, 1990). It is erroneous, however, to conclude that paid workers' labor power constitutes *in toto* the productive labor, or "health work," required to produce health care, social support, and long-term care services for the elderly.

Health Work Cost Management

Labor power has a value regardless of its concrete form and regardless of whether its owner chooses to sell his or her capacity to work. The rate of surplus value (the labor time performed solely for the capitalist or the rate of exploitation) is malleable, involves complex social relations of production, and can be increased by increasing worker productivity, decreasing worker pay, or adjusting the combination of paid workers to the lowest-cost combination that can produce the same output. The output is then relatively less costly and a portion (if not all) of the increased economic gain reverts to the capitalist system (or some may go to the suppliers of labor power, the workers, if they are successful in effectively negotiating that arrangement).

Work speedup and increased supervision are two management strategies that have been used to increase wage labor productivity in the home care industry (Szasz, 1990). A third strategy, adjusting the combination of paid workers to produce the same output for less cost by shifting as much work as possible to the least-skilled, and lowest-paid, health workers ("least-cost combination" of paid workers), is theoretically a finite resource to decrease labor costs. First, there is a practical limit to the least-expensive combination of paid workers that can effectively produce the same output. Second, regulatory mechanisms and licensure/certification constraints limit the type and extent to which such a strategy can be implemented. However, one possibility to procure labor power for no immediate cost is to engage "informal" workers to provide their labor power for no compensation. This labor, however, is not entirely "free" because its use necessarily implies a commodity transaction, effectively decreasing the supply of the commodity labor power in one market area while increasing the supply in another. It does have the instant advantage, however, of temporarily decreasing the cost for paid labor power.

Informalization of Health Work

During the Medicare post-PPS period, an enormous volume of health work shifted to outside of institutions and concomitantly to informal care providers in community settings, including the home

(Binney, Estes, & Humphers, 1993). The process of transferring care, "informalization," has two dimensions relevant to health work. The first involves transfer of selected services out of institutionally based systems such as hospitals and nursing homes into the noninstitutionally based provision arenas of home and community (Binney et al., 1993), relying on the labor of unpaid providers (usually family members or friends and usually women). The second aspect of informalization involves shifting "high-tech" procedures and complex medical care from paid workers in an institutional setting, such as the hospital, to paid workers in the home and community (Binney et al., 1993). Both informalization processes affect home care labor in several ways.

Reliance on the "informal" sector to provide care previously supplied by paid labor in institutions devalues the paid labor (in the general labor market) and effectively eliminates most employee-based governmental regulatory protection from the employer-worker-client relationship (Close, 1994). This has important consequences for both care providers and care recipients in areas such as worker's compensation for on-the-job injury and professional practice guidelines in negligent/abusive care situations. Another consequence of health care labor informalization is that it confounds accurate assessment of the actual supply, demand, and qualifications of labor needed for services provision (Close, 1994). Informalization allows for the use (and not coincidentally "consumption") of costly materials and equipment, without the costly investment of wages for the labor power required to provide these services. Informalization also directly and indirectly supports profits for organizations employing paid workers, such as those involved in the production of medications, equipment, supplies, and products used in the care of noninstitutionalized clients.

When informalization involves the shift from formal, institutionally based provider to formal, community-based provider, there is likely also a shift of high-tech, complex medical care from the hospital to the home (Binney et al., 1993). This situation poses numerous labor force quandaries, including questions of liability, training, supervision, and maintenance of the home-based, high-tech care system without the traditional institutionally based labor force resources supporting around-the-clock services of nurses, electrical technicians, environmental services, and substitute workers to cover breaks and meal times.

The process of informalization shifts caregiving responsibilities from paid to unpaid workers across the continuum of care. The results directly affect the formal-care workforce and associated labor market as well as the informal provider system. This topic is generally not problematized in the literature; rather, the vast and seemingly more fashionable debate over familial caregiving responsibility and burden usurps this discussion and tends to obfuscate broader structural issues such as the equitable distribution of care responsibilities by gender, race, and social class (Binney et al., 1993; Estes & Rundall, 1992), by individual, family, and society (Wolf, 1999), and the use of private versus public resources (Levine, 1999). The issue of informal health work is explicitly addressed in this chapter *because* it is becoming an implicit structural assumption in the health care cost containment debate and the policy strategies considered viable (Benjamin, 1993; Montgomery, 1999; Wood, 1991). Specifically, informal providers are expected to provide and maintain the home as a caregiving environment where unpaid workers conduct health work outside of costly institutions.

An enormous burden for care of homebound elderly rests with informal care providers. "Seventy percent of severely impaired elderly people rely solely on informal care from family and friends; only three percent rely exclusively on formal care" (Commonwealth Fund, 1989, p. 8; see also Chapters 6 and 10). In fact, the estimated variance associated with overall low use of only formal helpers among the frail elderly reported in National Long Term Care Surveys prevented analysts from estimating changes between 1982 and 1984 (National Center for Health Statistics [NCHS], 1993). Three of four informal caregivers are women, 80% of whom provide unpaid care 4 hours a day, 7 days a week (O'Rand & National Academy on Aging, 1994). Guralnik and Simonsick (1993) state that "almost no one with three or more ADLs can remain in the community with formal care only, that is, without the help of family and friends" (p. 7). The nearly $200 billion computed economic value of informal caregiving provided by 25.8 million caregivers who "work" without pay for 17.9 hours a week (Arno, Levine, & Memmott, 1999) substantiates the claim that there is a structural requirement for unpaid health workers to sustain the system of care outside of costly institutions.

From the standpoint of labor force and labor market issues relevant to the provision of care for older persons in the home, several observations about informal care are in order. Understudied and underdeveloped measures of workforce disruption associated with the phenomenon of women "responsible for" and actually providing the bulk of long-term care in homes prevent clear description and quantification of effects on the formal labor market (Estes & Close, 1994). Political rhetoric extolling the virtues of family (i.e., "free") caregiving persists. Notably few scholars or practitioners debate the questionable stance of public policy promoting informal care by embracing kinship obligation (Abel, 1995; Finch, 1989; Levine, 1999) as an appropriate social contract for provision of health and social services to older persons (Estes & Rundall, 1992; Phillipson, 1992). These factors contribute to issues of home care labor supply, worker qualifications, and education/training assuming a low priority in scholarly research and health care policy debates (Estes & Close, 1993).

Informal networks of family and friends provide approximately 80% to 90% of community-based long-term care (Stone, Cafferata, & Sangl, 1987). The exclusive use of formal care services is rare among older, impaired persons (Commonwealth Fund, 1988). The relationship between formal and informal care appears more complementary than substitutable (DeFriese & Woomert, 1992). It is well established that women are the major providers of informal, unpaid long-term care (Allen & Pifer, 1993). The combined effects of providing informal care and participating in the formal workforce can negatively affect the income, health, and emotional burden of female care providers (Abel, 1991; Allen & Pifer, 1993; Arendell & Estes, 1991). The consequences for adequate, safe care provision, as well as labor resources available in the formal sector, remain relatively uninvestigated. Regardless of any debate about whether care provision should be an individual's, a family's, or society's responsibility (Montgomery, 1999; Wolf, 1999), the necessity for human labor to provide care is indisputable.

Informal (unpaid) labor is rapidly becoming the hegemonic mainstay of health work provided to chronically disabled and acutely ill older persons. There is little dispute that current long-term care policy is built on the implicit assumption of informal care provision (see Chapter 6; Binney et al., 1993; Doty, 1995; Kapp, 1995; Montgomery, 1999). Informalization has the economic advantage of minimizing constant capital outlay as care moves from formal institutions to informal homes and community centers. There may also be political advantages to effectively obscuring public view of the workforce providing care and the conditions under which the care is provided. Informalization decreases direct costs associated with both constant and variable capital outlay. Less obvious are the ways in which informalization may affect indirect costs associated with the participation of informal care providers in the formal labor sector (specifically the participation of women in the paid labor force), the ability of paid home care workers to negotiate wages and benefits, the ability of demographers to accurately project health and long-term care worker supply and demand, and the influence of regulatory systems guaranteeing paid worker benefits and protections.

The increasing burden of home care for the informal provider system (the unpaid workers) is a frequently addressed issue in the literature. The major themes occurring in studies designed to describe and/or ameliorate caregiver "burden" (or "role strain" or "stress") tend to seek explanation for the family/individual sense of burden and to suggest/evaluate strategies—such as respite care and support groups for the caregiver—to support the caregiver in this continuing role. In contrast, relatively little literature critically analyzes the relationship between the formal and informal caregiving systems (Cancian & Oliker, 2000; Kempler, 1992; Soldo, Agree, & Wolf, 1989; Vaughan, 1997) and the potential for paying family members to provide in-home care (England, Linsk, Simon-Rusinowitz, & Keigher, 1990). No research appears to address the link between federal policy changes and unpaid workers in the home care environment; few studies have addressed the effects of policy changes on paid home care workers (Estes, Swan, & Associates, 1993; Szasz, 1990).

The impact of policy changes on the home care labor environment in the 1980s caused elevated workloads for paid workers who were increasingly monitored for productivity (Estes, 2000b; Estes, Swan, & Associates, 1993; Szasz, 1990). As the volume of work was burgeoning in the home care industry, cost containment policies restricted the options that agencies had available to increase wages and benefits (and still remain profitable) (Estes & Binney, 1997; Estes, Swan, & Associates, 1993; Szasz, 1990). As wages and benefits to paid workers were constrained in the Medicare-certified sector, competition for workers in the labor market should have grown, and there should have been a commensurate increase in the wages of home care workers. However, data indicate that wages for home care RNs, LVNs/LPNs, and home health aides remained significantly less than for workers in institutional settings (especially hospitals) in 1993 (National Association for Home Care [NAHC], 1993). The availability and systemic use of unpaid labor outside of institutions to perform the work that is performed by paid labor within institutions could partially account for this inconsistency. The "supply" of unfettered labor power in the home and community and the lack of regulatory oversight in private residences establishes an environment where unpaid, "unskilled," unlicensed, uncertified (however, quite possibly competent) workers provide the bulk of health work necessary to sustain service recipients outside of costly institutions.

Health Work Policy Environment: The Role of the State

Four major federal policy changes in the 1980s influenced health and long-term care labor in particular. The Omnibus Reconciliation Act of 1980 liberalized home health eligibility requirements and opened a wide path for the entrance of proprietary agencies into the home care business (Estes, Swan, Bergthold, & Spohn, 1992). The Medicare Prospective Payment System (1983), designed to contain spiraling hospital care costs by effectively shortening inpatient stays, literally pushed elderly (and others) out of institutions into the community-based long-term care system, causing a compensatory response in the system supplying health and social services to the elderly in their homes (Wood & Estes, 1990). This compensatory response involved the transformation of the home care industry reflected in the trend toward privatization, medicalization, and changes in labor conditions (Estes, Swan, & Associates, 1993). Organizational responses to these policy changes precipitated management strategies to alter the work process in attempts to maintain organizational viability and profit (Estes, Swan, & Associates, 1993; Szasz, 1990) by decreasing labor costs in the delivery of services.

The latter two policy changes were designed specifically with labor in mind as indicated in their explicit provisions. The 1987 Omnibus Budget Reconciliation Act (OBRA 1987) redefined the "homebound" eligibility requirement of Medicare and mandated minimum training requirements for paraprofessional long-term care workers in nursing homes and Medicare-certified home care agencies. In 1989, the Health Care Financing Administration (HCFA) clarified Medicare eligibility and coverage language, which effectively eased fiscal intermediaries' restrictive interpretation of the "part-time or intermittent" home health care benefit (Bishop & Skwara, 1993). An analysis of the effect of this interpretation indicates that overall growth in home health care from 1989 to 1992 was being driven by increasing average number of visits per beneficiary served as opposed to average charges per visit or an increase in the number of persons served (Bishop & Skwara, 1993).

The cost of home care labor could be decreased by changing the skill mix (and associated personnel costs) of the paid workers involved in the process of home care services delivery. However, federal regulations that limited the extent of skill mix adjustments within the paid labor sector (Szasz, 1990) also limited the utility of this maneuver. On the other hand, if a change in skill mix occurred across the paid-unpaid labor boundary, then regulatory constraint may not have been an obstacle to lowering agency labor costs by achieving less costly combinations of health workers (the paid and the unpaid).

Benjamin (1993) identifies early policy questions about the appropriateness of family care in the home that were generated by provider's concerns about training family members to render nursing and personal care services because of inconsistencies in educational level, language barriers, and cultural practices. These concerns have been neither adequately addressed in the literature nor publicly debated in any meaningful fashion. Reliance on the informal sector has apparently become a "given" constant in the home care labor equation. Wood (1991) argues that the burden of long-term care being borne by the family (female caregivers) helps control the public cost of long-term care and that this social arrangement is neither an appropriate nor a sustainable solution to the mounting challenge of providing long-term care. Levine (1999) encourages a new paradigm that considers patient, family, and professionals as a "complex and dynamic partnership." Consideration of the labor value invested by all members of this partnership would certainly help elucidate the "real costs" of home care (Kane, 1999).

Empirical evidence indicates that the vast majority of direct paid care for homebound elderly is being provided by personnel heavily representing the economic periphery (the home care aides and homemakers/chore workers) and by unpaid workers (mostly women) donating their labor power to health work in private residences (Gerstel & Gallagher, 1994). The location of home care in a service industry, specifically in the health care service industry, further embeds two unique characteristics of health care labor under capitalism: (a) dependency on the labor of women, minorities, and immigrants and (b) the increasing specialization and hierarchicalization of the health labor force (Navarro, 1986).

The labor needs of the rapidly expanding home care industry coupled with the structural reliance on the labor power of women, minorities, and immigrants foster the transfer of work from formal to informal providers. How might the requisite technical knowledge and skill be transferred to the informal providers? Recent investigation of Medicare-certified and uncertified home care agencies suggests that there exists a structural arrangement that fosters this transfer (Close, 1994; Estes & Swan, 1994). Analysis of home care agency requirements for the provision of "high-tech" care in the home indicates that the critical agency condition for patients to receive these services is the requirement for the patient/caregiver to be trained in the use of the technology. Furthermore, regardless of whether the home care agency required a primary caregiver, the implicit structural requirement for receipt of high-tech home care services was that unpaid labor power be invested in the process. Both Medicare-certified and uncertified agencies reported training paid personnel to train unpaid workers (patients, families, friends) who, in turn, then provided their uncompensated labor power to meet the home care agency requirement to receive high-tech care for the homebound elderly client (Close, 1994; Estes & Swan, 1994). Kane (1999) further explicates the targeting of home care according to the presence of informal caregivers.

Conclusion: A New Perspective on Health Work

In their discussion of the increasing demands placed on unpaid caregivers, Arendell and Estes (1991) identified four strategies women use to cope with the increasing burden of informal care. Three of the four strategies effectively involve systemic decreases in variable capital outlay for labor provided by women: specifically, caregiving women reduce their paid working hours, take time off without pay, or quit their jobs. Thus, to provide the "caregiving" (productive health work in home care), female caregivers may give up a portion or all of their wages and proceed to provide—or, more accurately, "donate"—their labor power for no compensation. Interestingly, evidence indicates that such caregiving does not necessarily interrupt women's wage labor, nor does employment preclude female caregiving responsibilities (Moen, Robison, & Fields, 1994). Recently, Kane (1999) amplified the need to clearly understand the distinction between "service" costs (formal sector only) and "real" costs (formal and informal sectors combined) when attempting to determine the relationship between effectiveness and costs of home care.

Any attempt to investigate, explain, or predict labor force needs for the delivery of health, social, and long-term care services outside of institutions is weakened by theoretical and practical disregard for the contribution of "free" labor power essential to the maintenance of service recipients in the community. Cancian and Oliker (2000) contend that this "devaluation of caregiving" relates to the perception of care as "a natural instinctual feminine activity" (Cancian & Oliker, 2000, p. 9). Care outside of formal institutions incurs less direct costs for agencies in both constant and variable capital outlays. The indirect costs, however, have important ramifications for (a) informal care providers' participation in the formal labor sector (specifically the participation of women in the paid labor force), (b) paid home care workers' negotiation of fair wages and benefits, (c) accurate projections of home care worker supply and demand, and (d) regulatory systems of worker benefits and protections as well as health worker and care recipient safety.

Because women, racial and ethnic minorities, and the elderly perform the great bulk of direct home care provision, the structural requirements for home care disproportionately affect those groups and simultaneously compromise their life course opportunities. In the past, this burden has been borne largely by the private sector. Increasing labor needs in the U.S. economy, increasing care needs of the rapidly expanding older generations, and the continuing policy disregard for the *real* labor inputs required for home care are on a crash course potentially deleterious to both the private and public sectors. Refusal to view health work as the combination of labor inputs provided by paid and unpaid workers "hides the costs of long-term care within the family domain and diverts attention from the problems of an inadequate formal care system by defining the problem as one of deficiency in the capacity and coping abilities of family caregivers" (Montgomery, 1999, p. 408).

Health work, particularly in home health care, involves a complex and interdependent array of labor inputs from both compensated and uncompensated workers. To understand the structural relationships necessary to provide adequate, cost-effective care in the future, society will need to more fully understand the intersection of formal and informal health work and recognize that both are economically and socially vital to planning for care needs.

Concluding Observations on Social Policy, Social Theory, and Research

Carroll L. Estes

This volume addresses the topic of social policy and aging. The theoretical framework and analytic approach is offered as a critical examination of policies and services for the aging in the United States.

Social Policy

A new level of ugly and unforgiving political partisanship over the past decade has engulfed social policy on aging as reflected in extremely intense power struggles over the two bedrock entitlement programs for the elderly—Social Security and Medicare. Empirical work in the social policy field during this period has been largely framed by the discipline of economics in case of Social Security and by the two disciplines of economics and medicine in the case of Medicare and health policy. The privatization of Social Security, in the context of the U.S. economy, the deficit reduction, and the demographic surge of the baby boomers, has been the predominant policy focus in aging that has consumed media and political attention throughout the 1990s (see

Chapter 5). In near mirror image is the call for Medicare reform via privatization strategies such as private insurance vouchers (see Chapters 3, 4, and 8).

The rhetoric of the privatization debate has incorporated and normalized the most conservative ideological vision of the neoliberal state (rather, antistate) by questioning the legitimacy and competence of the state, rather than the market, to meet the goals (economic security and health care) of these programs. The discourse of individual responsibility signals a disdainful rejection of a meaningful state role beyond one that promotes and funds market solutions while shifting responsibility away from the public or collective community and onto private individuals (see Chapter 9). The globalization of capital further extends the question of the respective roles of the state and the market. Indeed, there is debate about whether the state is "finished" or whether it is more important than ever in order to promote the further entrenchment and expansion of U.S. capitalism around the world.

The improving budget balance and rising surplus of the U.S. government in the last year of the Clinton presidency became a huge problem for conservative policymakers to manage, because they had, for two or more decades, constructed and used the federal deficit as the rationale to justify their efforts to diminish federal responsibility for the aged and to privatize both Social Security and Medicare. With regard to Social Security, larger questions of the "right" to entitlements or to any service or benefit as a U.S. citizen or immigrant are the subtext of the debate about the solvency of Social Security and proposals for a privatized system (see Chapter 5). Similar issues have dogged the Medicare program.

The critical perspective draws attention to conflicting power struggles over social policy and aging as these highlight the experience of "the citizen" and its meaning in the democratic state under U.S. and global capitalism (see Chapter 1). A major issue concerns new and critical thinking on the concept of citizenship (Sassoon, 1991), which acknowledges that treatment of individuals "as equals" under the law may well not deliver any form of substantive "equality" in the life experience of older persons, considering their varying attributes, situations, and social conditions. As Sassoon (1991) notes, "Differences between people according to resources and needs, family situation and point in life cycle, and life history with regard to the world of work are as significant as equality before the law or equal political rights" (p. 90).

This means that policymakers need to consider careful targeting of programs to achieve the desired *outcomes* of policy. The design of policies needs to go beyond merely being gender or race "neutral" in terms of the rules imposed to acknowledging that race, class, and gender differences make the policy outcomes for individuals unequal. Sassoon (1991) challenges the neoliberal notion of citizenship that rules out "the significance of difference ... while [citizenship] is posed as universal and abstract" (p. 95), as if the same law or policy creates the same result for individuals who are in vastly different circumstances. Sassoon argues that the "citizenry at large has a highly differentiated relationship to the state" (p. 98). This means that "on a concrete, practical level, equal achievement premised on integration into the dominant [citizen] model is impossible. Consequently these critiques assert the value and validity of different identities, or race, nationality, religion, gender" (p. 97). Claims of the universality of citizenship as an experience and reality obscure the inevitable imbalance of power (Sassoon, 1991) between individuals who are, in fact, situated in interlocking systems of oppression (Collins, 1990, 1991).

The critical perspective is sensitive to class, gender, and race/ethnicity and to the imperative consideration of structural or built-in forces such as institutional racism and sexism that contribute systemic barriers to fairness and equality of individual policy outcomes. The critical perspective promotes theory and methods that will illuminate these issues and investigate these barriers and their consequences for the health and economic security of older persons, while simultaneously drawing on a deep reservoir of sentiment that seeks to promote social justice in the everyday life of all older persons in the diverse society.

Social Theory and Research

Early chapters of this volume (see especially Chapters 2 and 3) point to what may be called an increasing theory-less empiricism and "social engineering" approach to social policy in aging as characterized by applied research on the demographics of aging, actuarial modeling and projections, the economics of aging, health, health care, and health financing that fails to measure (or to examine as problematic) either (a) the diverse experience of old age and aging or (b) the differential outcomes of social policy for the old in society, both of which are predictable and inevitable results of differences in their social location and which are profoundly influenced by race/ethnicity, class, and gender at both the individual and institutional levels. Often ignored are the complex results of the institutional processing and treatment through social policy across the life course in any particular socio-historical moment in time. As described in Chapter 3, the problems of aging for the individual and of the aging society tend to be defined as largely medical and amenable to technical correction within a paradigm predicated on the continued dominance of medicine and the commodification of the needs of the elderly.

A core feature of medical care commodification (see Chapters 3 and 8) is the definition of the needs of older people in terms of medical or other services and goods to be provided and "sold" for profit rather than thinking of such needs for services in terms of social need and the "right" of the elderly to economic and health security (Caplan, Light, & Daniels, 1999; Estes, Gerard, Zones, & Swan, 1984). There are serious implications for the nonprofit sector and the dimming of what remains of the altruistic residue there is in American society (see Chapter 4).

The current field of gerontological research surrounding social policy in many ways exemplifies social science "in the service of" reproducing the dominant institutions of society and the unequal distribution of power and material resources, thus perpetuating increasing inequality along the lines of the preexisting social divisions in society. Applications of the policy sciences to aging tend to take for granted the existing systems of medicine and capitalism as scholars work largely within "definitions of the situation" framed by economic paradigms, assumptions, and models of cost-effectiveness and individual-level outcomes. The end result is that such investigations consider only a limited array of potentially viable policy options, ensuring the serious consideration of only incremental changes that will do little to alter the basic condition of the elderly. There is a dearth of critical scholarship in the field, particularly in the discipline of economics itself (for an exception, see Rice, 1998). Examples are that research in health policy and aging takes for granted the assumptions underlying the market, as well as the validity of the theorized and "real" individual preferences and consumer "choices." Dominant economic interests and privilege are preserved by not examining as equally valid options the opposing thought structures of constructing and implementing other systems of governance that would promote a citizen right to the benefits of health and long-term care and to an adequate quality of life with economic security.

Challenging these approaches are political-economy theories, as well as critical, feminist, and cultural theories (see Chapters 1, 2, and 6). The substantial intellectual ferment in "the political economy of aging," "critical gerontology," and "humanistic gerontology" has resulted from a combination of, on the one hand, the infusion of theoretical developments in postmodernism, feminism, antiracist theory, critical theory, and cultural studies of science (Estes & Linkins, 1998; Moody, 1998; Phillipson, 1998) and, on the other hand, the challenge to the intellectual Left in the wake of the failure of communism, the gold rush of globalization concentrating heretofore unimaginable power and wealth in private hands, and the lack of what are perceived as viable socialist alternatives to the capitalist state. With the global market, the sovereignty of the nation-state is challenged as never before as "more and more of the national economy is owned by international corporations" (Turner, 1999, p. 274), which, in turn, raises more profound questions about the meaning of "the traditional forms of citizenship [that] . . . do not correspond to the idea of an increasingly global market" (p. 274).

These trends have fostered a great sense of urgency on two fronts: first, in the need to critically examine social policy and the welfare state at the institutional and world system level in ways that offer some hope of reclaiming or redeeming the citizen and the state from a social rights perspective (Kagarlitsky, 1999; Twine, 1994) and, second, in work challenging the dominant paradigms of knowledge construction. Some of the most important work in confronting scientific positivism has been contributed in the form of standpoint theory and feminist epistemology (Harding, 1996). This critique calls attention to the fact that in much mainstream research, women, minorities, and other disadvantaged groups and individuals "are routinely silenced or erased as actors in the production of . . . politics and policy" (Clarke & Olesen, 1999, p. 3)—and first and foremost, in the production of knowledge (Harding, 1996). This work challenges male biases and the lack of gendered and racial analyses in science. It seeks a retheorizing and revisioning or "letting go of how we have seen in order to construct new perceptions [that do not create] false universals that . . . erase significant differences" (Clarke & Olesen, 1999, p. 3), either between or within groups. "Knowledge of the empirical world is supposed to be grounded in [the] world (in complex ways). Human lives are part of the empirical world that scientists study; they are not homogeneous in any class, gender , or race-stratified society (Harding, 1996). The idea is that our conceptions of nature and the life sciences are "deeply social, historical and economic" in their construction (Clarke & Olesen, 1999, p. 9). It is the profound observation that, in one sense, nature does not exist outside of how we apprehend it and the way we see it, and that our way of seeing is not gender, class, and race blind. And it is a clarion call to provide empirically and theoretically better accounts generated from the perspective of the dominant ideology, which cannot see these conflicts and contradictions in the sex, gender or race/ethnicity systems as clues to the possibility of better explanations of nature and social life (Harding, 1996).

The critical perspective on social policy and aging challenges scholars to do the equivalent of what Gerda Lerner (1986) described as "stepping outside of patriarchal thought," which is being skeptical of known "systems of thought; being critical of all assumptions, ordering values and definitions" (Lerner, 1986, p. 228). It requires "trusting our own [diverse] . . . experience [even though] such experience has usually been trivialized or ignored [and] . . . means overcoming the deep-seated resistance within ourselves toward accepting ourselves and our knowledge as valid. . . . It means developing intellectual courage" (Lerner, 1986, p. 228).

There is a need for projects in the tradition of the Frankfurt School that are multidisciplinary and that examine the structural forces, "knowledges," and consciousness that profoundly shape social policy on old age and aging in any single society and in the global community of the first, second, and third worlds. Attention needs to be given to rebalancing studies of individual aging with research on the processing and treatment of the elderly in society, with emphasis on the "social," especially on the political, economic, and cultural conflicts and struggles that delineate the winners and losers of social policy. For it is social policy that sets the social provision and distribution of resources by the state and that materially affects the economic and health security of the different individuals and groups in the population across the life course.

Empirical and theoretical work on social policy and aging from a critical perspective opens the way for an alternative understanding and vision of "what is possible" for old age and aging. It is essential to lifting the ideological veil of scientific objectivity that obscures and mystifies inequality and social injustice in a society and economy that prioritizes the production of goods and services primarily (if not only) for its economic and exchange value rather than for its social value and capacity to meet human needs.

Required is a commitment not only to a reflexive social scientific approach to the study of social policy but also to praxis—that is, practice and social action that dialectically flow both from and into theory and research. At the level of praxis, the goal is to understand and change structures of dominance that produce and reproduce social inequality and injustice. Four interrelated dimensions of praxis are essential in the critical approach (Estes & Binney, 1989):

1. *The scientific,* giving attention to the situated nature of different knowledges and the influence of dominant theoretical and methodological approaches in shaping the research agenda and providing a partial (and occluded) view of the lives of the elderly and the potential policy options to meet their social needs

2. *The professional,* in specifying the power imbalances between elders and professionals and identifying their consequences for both recipients of care and their care providers

3. *Public policy,* in which the scientific work in gerontology and geriatrics itself is interrogated for how it shapes law and social policy based on the socially constructed "problems" of old age and the aging society

4. *Lay and public perceptions of old age and aging,* understood as a reflection of individual and group consciousness concerning what is appropriate responsibility for the state, the market, and the nonprofit sector and what is our individual and family responsibility for the aging and for the multiple generations implicated in how the society defines and treats the aging

The overall project of a critical perspective on social policy and aging is to provide alternative theoretical frameworks, a scientific epistemology, concrete information, and emancipatory knowledge that will contribute to a rebalancing of the imperatives of "the market" with the humanistic recognition and examination of the social threads that bind across generation, gender, race, ethnicity, and social class.

References

ABC News/*Washington Post* Poll. (1999). *Problems and priorities: Priorities for government.* Retrieved February 22, 2000, from PollingReport.com on the World Wide Web: pollingreport.com/prioriti.htm

Abel, E. K. (1986). The hospice movement: Institutionalizing innovation. *International Journal of Health Services, 16*(1), 71-85.

Abel, E. K. (1991). *Who cares for the elderly?* Philadelphia: Templeton University Press.

Abel, E. K. (1995). Man, woman, and chore boy? Transformation in the antagonistic demands of work and care on women in the nineteenth and twentieth centuries. *Milbank Quarterly, 74,* 187-211.

Abeles, R. P., Gift, H. C., & Ory, M. G. (1994). *Aging and quality of life.* New York: Springer.

Abramovitz, M. (1988). *Regulating the lives of women.* Boston: South End.

Abramson, A. J., & Salamon, L. M. (1986). *The nonprofit sector and the new federal budget.* Washington, DC: Urban Institute Press.

Acker, J. (1988). Class, gender and the relations of distribution. *Signs, 13*(3), 473-493.

Acker, J. (1992). Gendered institutions—From sex roles to gendered institutions. *Contemporary Sociology, 21,* 565-569.

Adler, N. E., Boyce, T., Chesney, M. A., Cohen, S., Folkman, S., Kahn, R. L., & Syme, S. L. (1994). Socioeconomic status and health: The challenge of the gradient. *American Psychologist, 49*(1), 15-24.

Adler, N. E., Boyce, W. T., Chesney, M. A., Folkman, S., & Syme, S. L. (1993). Socioeconomic inequalities in health: No easy solution. *Journal of the American Medical Association, 269*(24), 3140-3145.

Adler, N. E., & Coriell, M. (1997). Socioeconomic status and women's health. In S. J. Gallant, G. Puryear Keita, & R. Royak-Schaler (Eds.), *Health care for women: Psychological, social and behavioral influences* (pp. 11-23). Washington, DC: American Psychological Association.

Advisory Council on Social Security. (1997). *Report of the 1994-1996 Advisory Council on Social Security: Vol. 1. Findings and recommendations.* Washington, DC: Author.

Alford, R. R. (1975). *Health care politics: Ideological and interest group barriers to reform.* Chicago: University of Chicago Press.

Alford, R. R. (1992). The political language of the nonprofit sector. In R. M. Merelman (Ed.), *Language, symbolism, and politics* (pp. 17-50). Boulder, CO: Westview.

Alford, R. R., & Friedland, R. (1985). *Powers of theory: Capitalism, the state, and democracy.* New York: Cambridge University Press.

Allen, J., & Pifer, J. (Eds.). (1993). *Women on the front lines: Meeting the challenges of an aging America.* Washington, DC: Urban Institute.

American Association of Fund-Raising Counsel. (1989). *AAFRC trust for philanthropy* (annual report). New York: Giving USA.

American Association of Retired Persons. (1994). *The cost of long term care* (Fact Sheet No. 14-R). Washington, DC: Author.

American Association of Retired Persons, & Lewin Group. (1997). *Out-of-pocket health spending by beneficiaries age 65 and older* (Report 9704). Washington, DC: Public Policy Institute.

American Council on Life Insurance. (1998). *Who will pay for the baby boomers' long term care needs? Expanding the role of private long term care insurance.* Washington, DC: Author.

American Hospital Association. (1989). *Hospital statistics* (1989-1990 edition). Chicago: Author.

American Hospital Association. (1996). *Hospital statistics* (1996-1997 edition). Chicago: Author.

American Hospital Association. (1997). *AHA guide to the health care field* (1997-1998). Chicago: Author.

Amick, B. C., Levine, S., Tarlov, A. R., & Walsh, D. C. (1995). Introduction. In B. C. Amick, S. Levine, A. R. Tarlov, & D. C. Walsh (Eds.), *Society & health* (pp. 3-17). New York: Oxford University Press.

Andersen, R. M., & Mullner, R. M. (1989). Trends in the organization of health services. In H. E. Freeman & S. Levine (Eds.), *Handbook of medical sociology* (4th ed., pp. 144-165). Englewood Cliffs, NJ: Prentice Hall.

Anderson, R. N. (1998). United States abridged life tables, 1996. *National Vital Statistics Reports* (Vol. 47, No. 13). Hyattsville, MD: National Center for Health Statistics.

Andrews, C. (1995). *Profit fever: The drive to corporatize health care and how to stop it.* Monroe, ME: Common Courage Press.

Antonovsky, A. (1967). Social class, life expectancy and overall mortality. *Milbank Memorial Fund Quarterly/Health and Society, 45,* 31-73.

Arato, A., & Gebhardt, E. (1982). *Essential Frankfurt School reader.* New York: Continuum.

Arendell, T., & Estes, C. L. (1991). Older women in the post-Reagan era. *International Journal of Health Services, 21*(1), 59-73.

Arluke, A., & Peterson, J. (1981). Accidental medicalization of old age and its social control implications. In C. L. Frye (Ed.)., *Dimension: Aging, culture, and health.* Brooklyn, NY: J. F. Bergen.

Arno, P. S., Levine, C., & Memmott, M. M. (1999). The economic value of informal caregiving. *Health Affairs, 18*(2), 182-188.

Aspen Institute. (1998, November). *Health care conversions and philanthropy.* Paper presented at the Conference of the California Nonprofit Research Program of the Nonprofit Research Fund, San Francisco.

Baars, J. (1991). The challenge of critical gerontology: The problem of social constitution. *Journal of Aging Studies, 5*(3), 219-243.

Baker, D. (1999, May/June). Misleading options on Social Security. *Extra!,* p. 15.

Baker, D., & Weisbrot, M. (1999). *Social Security: The phony crisis.* Chicago: University of Chicago Press.

Balbo, L. (1982). The servicing work of women and the capitalist state. *Political Power & Social Theory, 3,* 251-270.

Ball, R. M. (1981). Rethinking national policy on health care for the elderly. In A. R. Somers & D. R. Fabian (Eds.), *The geriatric imperative.* New York: Appleton-Century-Crofts.

Baltes, P. B., & Baltes, M. M. (1990). *Successful aging: Perspectives from the behavioral sciences.* New York: Cambridge University Press.

Bass, S. A., Caro, F. G., & Chen, Y. P. (Eds.). (1993). *Achieving a productive aging society* (pp. 21-38). Westport, CT: Auburn House.

Bell, D. (1976). *The cultural contradictions of capitalism.* New York: Basic Books.

Bellandi, D., & Jaspen, B. (1998, May 25). While you weren't sleeping. *Modern Healthcare,* 35-42.

Belloc, N. B., & Breslow, L. (1972). Relationship of physical health status and health practices. *Preventive Medicine, 1,* 409-421.

Bengtson, V. L., Burgess, E. O., & Parrott, T. M. (1997). Theory, explanation, and a third generation of theoretical development in social gerontology. *Journal of Gerontology: Series B, Psychological Sciences and Social Sciences, 52*(2), S72-S88.

Bengtson, V. L., & Schaie, K. W. (Eds.). (1999). *Handbook of theories of aging.* New York: Springer.

Benjamin, A. E. (1993). A historical perspective on home care policy. *Milbank Quarterly, 71,* 129-166.

Berger, P. L., & Luckmann, T. (1966). *The social construction of reality: A treatise in the sociology of knowledge.* Garden City, NY: Doubleday.

Bergthold, L. (1990). *Purchasing power in health: Business, the state, and health care politics.* New Brunswick, NJ: Rutgers University Press.

Bergthold, L. A., Estes, C. L., & Villanueva, A. (1990). Public light and private dark: The privatization of home health services for the elderly in the United States. *Home Health Services Quarterly, 11*(3-4), 7-33.

Berkman, L. F., & Breslow, L. (1983). *Health and ways of living: The Alameda County study.* New York: Oxford University Press.

Berkman, L. F., & Syme, S. L. (1979). Social networks, host resistance, and mortality: A nine-year follow-up study of Alameda County residents. *American Journal of Epidemiology, 109*(2), 186-204.

Berliner, H. S., & Burlage, R. K. (1990). Proprietary hospital chains and academic medical centers. In J. W. Salmon (Ed.), *The corporate transformation of health care: Issues and directions* (pp. 97-116). Amityville, NY: Baywood.

Berliner, H. S., & Regan, C. (1990). Multi-national operations of U.S. for profit hospital chains: Trends and implications. In J. W. Salmon (Ed.), *The corporate transformation of health care: Issues and directions* (pp. 155-165). Amityville, NY: Baywood.

Bierstedt, R. (1964). Legitimacy. In J. Gould & W. L. Kolb (Eds.), *A dictionary of the social sciences* (pp. 386-387). New York: Free Press.

Biggs, S. (1997). Choosing not to be old? Masks, bodies and identity management in later life. *Ageing and Society, 17*(5), 553-570.

Binney, E. A., Estes, C. L., & Humphers, S. E. (1993). Informalization and community care. In C. L. Estes, J. H. Swan, & associates (Eds.), *The long term care crisis: Elders trapped in the No-care Zone* (pp. 155-170). Newbury Park, CA: Sage.

Binney, E. A., Estes, C. L., & Ingman, S. R. (1990). Medicalization, public-policy and the elderly: Social-services in jeopardy? *Social Science & Medicine, 30*(7), 761-771.

Bishop, C., & Skwara, K. C. (1993). Recent growth of Medicare home health. *Health Affairs, 12*(3), 95-110.

Black, D., Townsend, P., & Davidson, N. (1982). *Inequalities and health: The Black report.* Harmondsworth, UK: Penguin.

Blowing the whistle on Columbia/HCA: An interview with Marc Gardner. (1998, April). *Multinational Monitor, 19,* 17-20.

Bond, P., & Weissman, R. (1997). The costs of mergers and acquisitions in the U.S. health care sector. *International Journal of Health Services, 27*(1), 77-87.

Bortz, W. M., 3rd, & Bortz, W. M., 2nd. (1996). How fast do we age? Exercise performance over time as a biomarker. *Journal of Gerontology: Series A, Biological Sciences and Medical Sciences, 51*(5), M223-M225.

Bottomore, T. B. (1983). *A dictionary of Marxist thought.* Cambridge, MA: Harvard University Press.

Bound, J., Duncan, G. J., Laren, D. S., & Oleinick, L. (1991). Poverty dynamics in widowhood. *Journal of Gerontology, 46*(3), S115-S124.

Braden, B. R., Cowan, C. A., Lazenby, H. C., Martin, A. B., McDonnell, P. A., Sensenig, A. L., Stiller, J. M., Whittle, L. S., Donham, C. S., Long, A. M., & Stewart, M. W. (1998). National health expenditures, 1997. *Health Care Financing Review, 20*(1), 83-126.

Braverman, H. (1974). *Labor and monopoly capital: The degradation of work in the twentieth century.* New York: Monthly Review Press.

Brotman, H. B. (1982). *Every ninth American.* Washington, DC: U.S. Government Printing Office.

Brown, R. S., Clement, D. G., Hill, J. W., Retchin, S. M., & Bergeron, J. W. (1993). Do health maintenance organizations work for Medicare? *Health Care Financing Review, 15*(1), 7-23.

Brown, W. (1995). *States of injury: Power and freedom in late modernity.* Princeton, NJ: Princeton University Press.

Bunker, J. P., Gomby, D. S., & Kehrer, B. H. (Eds.). (1989). *Pathways to health: The role of social factors.* Menlo Park, CA: Henry J. Kaiser Family Foundation.

Burbridge, L. C. (1993). The labor market for home care workers: Demand, supply, and institutional barriers. *The Gerontologist, 33,* 41-46.

Burggraf, S. P. (1997). *The feminine economy and economic man: Reviving the role of family in the post-industrial age.* Reading, MA: Addison-Wesley.

Burkhauser, R. V., & Smeeding, T. M. (1994). *Social Security reform: A budget neutral approach to reducing older women's disproportionate risk of poverty* (Policy Brief 2). Syracuse, NY: Maxwell School Center for Policy Research.

Butler, L. H., & Newacheck, P. W. (1981). Health and social factors affecting long-term care policy. In J. Meltzer, F. Farrow, & H. Richman (Eds.), *Policy options in long-term care.* Chicago: University of Chicago Press.

Butler, R. N. (1996). On behalf of older women. Another reason to protect Medicare and Medicaid. *New England Journal of Medicine, 334*(12), 794-796.

Butler, R. N., & Lewis, M. I. (1982). *Aging and mental health* (3rd ed.). St. Louis, MO: Mosby.

Butler, R. N., & Schechter, M. (1995). Productive aging. In G. L. Maddox (Ed.), *The encyclopedia of aging: A comprehensive resource in gerontology and geriatrics.* New York: Springer.

Calasanti, T., & Zajicek, A. (1993). A socialist feminist approach to aging: Embracing diversity. *Journal of Aging Studies, 7*(2), 117-131.

Calasanti, T. M. (1993). Introduction: A socialist-feminist approach to aging. *Journal of Aging Studies, 7*(2), 107-109.

Calasanti, T. M. (1996). Incorporating diversity: Meaning, levels of research, and implications for theory. *The Gerontologist, 36*(2), 147-156.

California Association of Hospitals and Health Systems. (1988). Conversions. *News, 20*(25).

Cancian, F. M., & Oliker, S. J. (2000). *Caring and gender.* Thousand Oaks, CA: Pine Forge.

Cantor, M., & Little, V. (1985). Aging and social care. In R. H. Binstock & E. Shanas (Eds.), *Handbook of aging and the social sciences* (pp. 745-781). New York: Van Nostrand Reinhold.

Caplan, R. L., Light, D. W., & Daniels, N. (1999). Benchmarks of fairness: A moral framework for assessing equity. *International Journal of Health Services, 29*(4), 853-869.

Carrasquillo, O., Himmelstein, D., Woolhandler, S., & Bor, D. (1999). Going bare: Trends in health insurance coverage, 1989-1996. *American Journal of Public Health, 89*, 36-42.

Castells, M. (1989). *The informational city: Information technology, economic restructuring, and the urban-regional process.* Cambridge, MA: Basil Blackwell.

CBS News Poll. (2000). *Priorities for government: Poll, February 6-10, 2000.* Retrieved February 22, 2000, from PollingReport.com on the World Wide Web: pollingreport. com/prioriti.htm

Center on Budget and Policy Priorities. (1999). *The state fiscal analysis initiative (SFAI): Building organizational capacity for state budget and tax analysis.* Washington, DC: Author.

Chafetz, J. S. (1997). Feminist theory and sociology: Underutilized contributions for mainstream theory. *Annual Review of Sociology, 23*, 97-120.

Chernomas, R. (1999). Inequality as a basis for the U.S. emergence from the great stagnation. *International Journal of Health Services, 29*(4), 821-832.

Clark, R., & Spengler, J. (1980). *The economics of individual and population aging.* London: Cambridge University Press.

Clarke, A., & Olesen, V. (1999). Revising, diffracting, acting. In A. Clarke & V. Olesen (Eds.), *Revisioning women, health and healing* (pp. 3-48). New York: Routledge.

Clements, J. (1990, January 8). Insurance. *Forbes*, pp. 184-186.

Close, E. L. (1994). *A political economy perspective on home care labor.* Unpublished doctoral dissertation, University of California, San Francisco.

CNN/*Time* Poll. (1998). *What do you think is the single most important problem for the government to address in the coming year? Poll, June 30-July 1, 1998.* Retrieved July 9, 1998, from PollingReport.com on the World Wide Web: pollingreport.com/issues.htm

Coburn, D. (1999). Phases of capitalism, welfare states, medical dominance, and health care in Ontario. *International Journal of Health Services, 29*(4), 833-851.

Cole, T., Achenbaum, A., Jakobi, P., & Kastenbaum, R. (Eds.). (1993). *Voices and visions of aging: Toward a critical gerontology.* New York: Springer.

Cole, T. R. (1992). *The journey of life: a cultural history of aging in America.* New York: Cambridge University Press.

Coleman, B. J. (1998). *New directions for state long-term care systems* (2nd ed.). Washington, DC: Public Policy Institute, American Association of Retired Persons.

Collins, C. A., & Williams, D. R. (1999). Segregation and mortality: The deadly effects of racism? *Sociological Forum, 14,* 495-523.

Collins, P. H. (1990). *Black feminist thought: Knowledge, consciousness, and the politics of empowerment.* Boston: Unwin-Hyman.

Collins, P. H. (1991). *Black feminist thought: Knowledge, consciousness, and the politics of empowerment.* New York: Routledge.

Collins, R. (1988). *Theoretical sociology.* San Diego, CA: Harcourt Brace Jovanovich.

Commonwealth Fund. (1987). *Medicare's poor: Filling the gaps in medical coverage for low-income elderly Americans* (Report of the Commonwealth Fund Commission on Elderly People Living Alone). New York: Author.

Commonwealth Fund. (1988). *Aging alone: Profiles and projections* (Report of the Commonwealth Fund Commission on Elderly People Living Alone). New York: Author.

Commonwealth Fund. (1989). *Help at home: Long-term care assistance for impaired elderly people* (Report of the Commonwealth Fund Commission on Elderly People Living at Home). New York: Author.

Condon, B. (1998, January 12). Health care products. *Forbes,* pp. 176-178.

Connell, R. W. (1987). *Gender and power: Society, the person, and sexual politics.* Stanford, CA: Stanford University Press.

Conrad, P., & Schneider, J. W. (1992). *Deviance and medicalization: From badness to sickness* (Rev. ed.). Philadelphia: Temple University Press.

Cook, F. L. (1998, November 22). *The new politics of Social Security.* Paper presented at the annual meeting of the Gerontological Society of America, Philadelphia.

Costa, P. T., & McCrae, R. R. (1980). Still stable after all these years. In P. B. Baltes & O. G. Brim (Eds.), *Life-span development and behavior* (Vol. 3, pp. 65-102). New York: Academic Press.

Cryan, M. A., & Gardner, P. (1999). *Balancing mission and market: Nonprofits walk a tightrope between the public and private spheres.* San Francisco: Consumers Union, West Coast Regional Office.

Crystal, S. (1982). *America's old age crisis.* New York: Basic Books.

Crystal, S., & Shea, D. (1990). Cumulative advantage, cumulative disadvantage, and inequality among elderly people. *The Gerontologist, 30*(4), 437-443.

Crystal, S., & Waehrer, K. (1996). Later-life economic inequality in longitudinal perspective. *Journal of Gerontology: Series B, Psychological Sciences and Social Sciences, 51*(6), S307-S318.

Cumming, E., & Henry, W. E. (1961). *Growing old: The process of disengagement.* New York: Basic Books.

Dalaker, J., & Naifeh, M. (1997). *Poverty in the United States* (Current population reports, Series P60-201). Washington, DC: U.S. Government Printing Office.

Dannefer, D., & Uhlenberg, P. (1999). Paths of the life course: A typology. In V. L. Bengtson & K. W. Schaie (Eds.), *Handbook of theories of aging* (pp. 306-326). New York: Springer.

Davis, K. (1985). Equal treatment and unequal benefits: The Medicare program. *Milbank Memorial Fund Quarterly/Health and Society, 54*(4), 449-488.

DeFriese, G. H., & Woomert, A. (Eds.). (1992). *Informal and formal health care systems serving older persons.* Newbury Park, CA: Sage.

DePearl, N. A. M. (1999, February). *The future of Medicare.* Paper presented at the Commonwealth Fund Conference on the Future of Medicare, Washington, DC.

De Vita, C. (1997). *Viewing nonprofits across the states.* Washington, DC: Urban Institute.

Dews, P., & Habermas, J. (1986). *Autonomy and solidarity: Interviews with Jürgen Habermas.* London, UK: Verso.

Diamond, T. (1992). *Making gray gold: Narratives of nursing home care.* Chicago: University of Chicago Press.

Dickinson, J., & Russell, B. (1986). *Family, economy & state: The social reproduction process under capitalism.* New York: St. Martin's.

DiMaggio, P., & Powell, W. (1983). The iron cage revisited: Institutional isomorphism and collective rationality in organization fields. *American Sociological Review, 82,* 147-160.

Disability Rights Advocates. (1997). *Disability watch: The status of people with disabilities in the US.* Volcano, CA: Volcano Press.

Doty, P. (1995). Family caregiving and access to publicly funded home care. In R. A. Kane & J. D. Penrod (Eds.), *Family caregiving in an aging society* (pp. 92-122). Thousand Oaks, CA: Sage.

Dressel, P. L. (1988). Gender, race, and class: Beyond the feminization of poverty in later life. *The Gerontologist, 28*(2), 177-180.

Dressel, P. M., Minkler, M., & Yen, I. (1999). Gender, race, class and aging: Advances and opportunities. In M. Minkler & C. L. Estes (Eds.), *Critical gerontology: Perspectives from political and moral economy* (pp. 275-294). Amityville, NY: Baywood.

Dube, M. (1999, January). Lighten your load: In the race to compete, public hospitals shed excess baggage. *Trustee,* pp. 17-19.

Dubos, R. (1979). *Mirage of health.* New York: Harper & Row.

Edelman, M. (1964). *The symbolic uses of politics.* Urbana: University of Illinois Press.

Egan, A. H. (2000, July). *New Mexico civil society and devolution: Assets, contradictions and challenges.* Paper presented at the International Society for Third Sector Research, Dublin, Ireland.

Egan, A. H., & Shaening, M. (1996). *Medicaid managed care for behavioral health services in New Mexico: Recommendations for structuring a carve-out system.* Report to New Mexico Department of Health, Santa Fe.

Ehrenreich, B., & Ehrenreich, J. (1971). *The American health empire: Power, profits, and politics* (Report for the Health Policy Advisory Center [Health-PAC]). New York: Vintage.

Ehrenreich, J., & Ehrenreich, B. (1978). Medicine and social control. In J. Ehrenreich (Ed.), *The cultural crisis of modern medicine* (pp. 39-79). New York: Monthly Review Press.

Elder, G., Jr. (1992). Essay on the life course. In M. L. Borgatta & E. F. Borgatta (Eds.), *Encyclopedia of sociology* (pp. 1120-1130). New York: Macmillan.

England, S. E., Linsk, N. I., Simon-Rusinowitz, L., & Keigher, S. M. (1990). Paying kin for care: Agency barriers to formalizing informal care. *Journal of Aging and Social Policy, 2,* 63-86.

Ermann, D., & Gabel, J. (1984). Multihospital systems: Issues and empirical findings. *Health Affairs, 3*(1), 50-64.

Esping-Andersen, G. (1990). *The three worlds of welfare capitalism.* Cambridge, UK: Polity.

Estes, C. L. (1972). *Community planning for the elderly from an organizational, political, and interactionist perspective.* Unpublished doctoral dissertation, University of California, San Diego.

Estes, C. L. (1979). *The aging enterprise.* San Francisco: Jossey-Bass.

Estes, C. L. (1980). Constructions of reality. *Journal of Social Issues, 36*(2), 117-132.

Estes, C. L. (1981). The social construction of reality: A framework for inquiry. In P. R. Lee, N. B. Ramsay, & I. Red (Eds.), *The nation's health* (pp. 395-402). San Francisco: Boyd & Fraser.

Estes, C. L. (1982). Austerity and aging in the United States: 1980 and beyond. *International Journal of Health Services, 12*(4), 573-584.

Estes, C. L. (1983). Social Security: The social construction of a crisis. *Milbank Memorial Fund Quarterly/Health and Society, 61*(3), 445-461.

Estes, C. L. (1986a). The aging enterprise: In whose interests? *International Journal of Health Services, 16*(2), 243-251.

Estes, C. L. (1986b). The politics of aging in America. *Ageing and Society, 6,* 121-134.

Estes, C. L. (1991a). The new political economy of aging: Introduction and critique. In M. Minkler & C. L. Estes (Eds.), *Critical perspectives on aging: The political and moral economy of growing old* (pp. 19-36). Amityville, NY: Baywood.

Estes, C. L. (1991b). The Reagan legacy: Privatization, the welfare state, and aging in the 1990's. In J. Myles & J. S. Quadagno (Eds.), *States, labor markets, and the future of old age policy* (pp. 59-83). Philadelphia: Temple University Press.

Estes, C. L. (1993). The aging enterprise revisited. *The Gerontologist, 33*(3), 292-298.

Estes, C. L. (1996, November). *Crisis, the welfare state and aging* (Presidential address). Paper presented at the Annual Meeting of the Gerontological Society of America, Washington, DC.

Estes, C. L. (1998a, February). *Older women and the welfare state.* Keynote address at the Conference on Autonomy and Aging, Kingston University, Kingston-upon-Thames, UK.

Estes, C. L. (1998b, July). *Patriarchy and the welfare state revisited: The state, gender and aging.* Paper presented at the World Congress of Sociology, Montreal, Canada.

Estes, C. L. (1999a). Critical gerontology and the new political economy of aging. In M. Minkler & C. L. Estes (Eds.), *Critical gerontology: Perspectives from political and moral economy* (pp. 17-35). Amityville, NY: Baywood.

Estes, C. L. (1999b, April). *Moral economy, crisis, the welfare state, and aging: Toward cultural gerontology.* Invited lecture, Berlin, Germany.

Estes, C. L. (2000a). The political economy of aging. In G. Maddox (Ed.), *The encyclopedia of aging.* New York: Springer.

Estes, C. L. (2000b, April). The uncertain future of home care. In R. Binstock & L. Cluff (Eds.), *Home care advances: Essential research and policy issues* (pp. 239-253). New York: Springer.

Estes, C. L., & Alford, R. R. (1990). Systemic crisis and the nonprofit sector: Toward a political economy of the nonprofit health and social services sector. *Theory and Society, 19*(2), 173-198.

Estes, C. L., Alford, R. R., & Binney, E. A. (1987). *Restructuring the nonprofit sector.* San Francisco: University of California, Institute for Health and Aging.

Estes, C. L., & Bergthold, L. A. (1989). The unraveling of the nonprofit service sector in the U.S. *International Journal of Sociology and Social Policy, 9*(213), 18-33.

Estes, C. L., & Binney, E. A. (1988). Toward a transformation of health and aging policy. *International Journal of Health Services, 18*(1), 69-82.

Estes, C. L., & Binney, E. A. (1989). The biomedicalization of aging: Dangers and dilemmas. *The Gerontologist, 29*(5), 587-596.

Estes, C. L., & Binney, E. A. (1990). *Older women and the state.* Unpublished manuscript. San Francisco: University of California, Institute for Health and Aging.

Estes, C. L., & Binney, E. A. (1993). Restructuring the nonprofit sector. In C. L. Estes, J. H. Swan, & associates (Eds.), *The long-term care crisis: Elders trapped in the no-care zone* (pp. 22-42). Newbury Park, CA: Sage.

Estes, C. L., & Binney, E. A. (1997). The restructuring of home care. In D. M. Fox & C. Raphael (Eds.), *Home based care for a new century* (pp. 5-21). Cambridge, MA: Basil Blackwell.

Estes, C. L., Binney, E. A., & Bergthold, L. (1989a). How the legitimacy of the sector has eroded. In V. A. Hodgkinson & R. W. Lyman (Eds.), *The future of the nonprofit sector: Challenges, changes, and policy considerations,* (pp. 21-40). San Francisco: Jossey-Bass.

Estes, C. L., Binney, E. A., & Bergthold, L. (1989b). The role of ideology and public policy: The deligitimation of the nonprofit sector. In V. A. Hodgkinson & R. W. Lyman (Eds.), *The future of the nonprofit sector: Challenges, changes, and policy considerations* (pp. 21-40). San Francisco: Jossey-Bass.

Estes, C. L., Binney, E. A., & Culbertson, R. A. (1992). The gerontological imagination: Social influences on the development of gerontology, 1945-present. *International Journal of Aging and Human Development, 35*(1), 49-65.

Estes, C. L., & Close, L. (1993). *Long-term care: The challenge to education* (The Beverly Lecture on Gerontology and Geriatrics Education, No. 8). Washington, DC: Association for Gerontology in Higher Education.

Estes, C. L., & Close, L. (1994). Public policy and long-term care. In R. P. Abeles, H. C. Gift, & M. G. Ory (Eds.), *Aging and quality of life* (pp. 310-335). New York: Springer.

Estes, C. L., Gerard, L., & Clarke, A. (1984). Women and the economics of aging. *International Journal of Health Services, 14*(1), 55-68.

Estes, C. L., Gerard, L., Zones, J. S., & Swan, J. (1984). *Political economy, health, and aging.* Boston: Little Brown.

Estes, C. L., Harrington, C., & Davis, S. (1992). Medical industrial complex. In M. L. Borgatta & E. F. Borgatta (Eds.), *Encyclopedia of sociology* (pp. 1243-1254). New York: Macmillan.

Estes, C. L., Harrington, C., & Pellow, D. (2000). The medical industrial complex. In E. Borgatta & M. Borgatta (Eds.), *The encyclopedia of sociology* (2nd ed., Vol. 2) (pp. 136-148). New York: Macmillan.

Estes, C. L., & Linkins, K. W. (1997). Devolution and aging policy: Racing to the bottom in long-term care. *International Journal of Health Services, 27*(3), 427-442.

Estes, C. L., & Linkins, K. W. (1998). Decentralization, devolution, and the deficit: The changing role of the state and the community. In J. G. Gonya (Ed.), *Resecuring Social Security and Medicare: Understanding privatization and risk* (pp. 37-44). Washington, DC: Gerontological Society of America.

Estes, C. L., Linkins, K. W., & Binney, E. A. (1996). The political economy of aging. In R. H. Binstock & L. K. George (Eds.), *Handbook of aging and the social sciences* (pp. 346-361). San Diego, CA: Academic Press.

Estes, C. L., Linkins, K. W., Lynch, M., Newcomer, R. J., Rice, D., & Rummelsberg, J. (1998). *Trends, issues and assumptions related to the future of health and health care for the elderly* (Report prepared for the Institute for the Future). San Francisco: University of California, Institute for Health & Aging.

Estes, C. L., & Mahoney, C. (1986, March). *Philanthropy, nonprofits, and health policy* (panel presentation). Presented at the annual conference of the Independent Sector, Public Policy Among Subsectors, Chicago.

Estes, C. L., & Michel, M. (1999). Social Security and women. In America Task Force on Women (Ed.), *Social Security in the 21st century*. Washington, DC: Gerontological Society of America.

Estes, C. L., & Rundall, T. G. (1992). Social characteristics, social structures, and health in the aging population. In M. G. Ory, R. P. Abeles, & E. Darby (Eds.), *Aging, health, and behavior* (pp. 299-326). Newbury Park, CA: Sage.

Estes, C. L., & Swan, J. H. (1994). Privatization, system membership, and access to home health care for the elderly. *Milbank Quarterly, 72*(2), 277-298.

Estes, C. L., Swan, J. H., & associates. (1993). *The long-term care crisis: Elders trapped in the no-care zone*. Newbury Park, CA: Sage.

Estes, C. L., Swan, J. H., Bergthold, L. A., & Spohn, P. H. (1992). Running as fast as they can: Organizational changes in home health care. *Home Health Care Services Quarterly, 13*(1-2), 35-69.

Estes, C. L., Swan, J. H., & Gerard, L. (1982). Dominant and competing paradigms: Toward a political economy of aging. *Ageing and Society, 2*(2), 151-164.

Estes, C. L., Wallace, S. P., & Linkins, K. W. (2000). Political economy of health and aging. In C. E. Bird, P. Conrad, & A. M. Fremont (Eds.), *Handbook of medical sociology* (5th ed., pp. 129-142). Upper Saddle River, NJ: Prentice Hall.

Estes, C. L., & Weitz, T. A. (2000). Aging and gender: A new voice on the women's health agenda. In P. R. Lee & C. L. Estes (Eds.), *The nation's health* (6th ed.) (pp. 523-546). Boston: Jones & Bartlett.

Estes, C. L., Wiener, J. M., Goldberg, S. C., & Goldensen, S. M. (2000). The politics of long term care reform under the Clinton health plan: Lessons for the future. In P. R. Lee & C. L. Estes (Eds.), *The nation's health* (6th ed.) (pp. 206-214). Boston, MA: Jones & Bartlett.

Estes, C. L., & Wood, J. B. (1986). The nonprofit sector and community-based care for the elderly in the United States: A disappearing resource. *Social Science & Medicine, 23*(12), 1261-1266.

Evashwick, C. J., Rundall, T., & Goldiamond, B. (1985). Hospital services for older adults. *The Gerontologist, 25*(6), 631-637.

Farrand, M. (1999, May/June). Social Security coverage: By the numbers. *Extra!* p. 9.

Feder, J. (2000, April). *Covering the uninsured: The difference different proposals make.* Paper presented at the Dorothy Peckman Rice Symposium, San Francisco.

Federation of American Health Systems. (1990). *Federation of American Health Systems* (1990 Directory). Little Rock, AR.

Feinstein, J. S. (1993). The relationship between socioeconomic status and health: A review of the literature. *Milbank Quarterly, 71*(2), 279-322.

Feldman, J. J., Makuc, D. M., Kleinman, J. C., & Cornoni-Huntley, J. (1989). National trends in educational differentials in mortality. *American Journal of Epidemiology, 129*(5), 919-933.

Feldstein, P. J. (1988). *Health care economics.* New York: John Wiley.

Feldstein, P. J. (1993). *Home care economics* (4th ed.). New York: John Wiley.

Ferraro, K. F., & Farmer, M. M. (1996). Double jeopardy, aging as leveler, or persistent health inequality? A longitudinal analysis of white and black Americans. *Journals of Gerontology: Series B, Psychological Sciences and Social Sciences, 51*(6), S319-S328.

Finch, J. (1989). *Family obligations and social change.* London: Polity Press & Basil Blackwell.

Finch, J., & Groves, D. (1983). *A labour of love: Women, work, and caring.* London: Routledge & Kegan Paul.

Firestone, S. (1970). *The dialectic of sex: The case for feminist revolution.* New York: William Morrow.

Firestone, S. (1979). *The dialectic of sex: The case for feminist revolution* (Reprint ed.). London: Women's Press.

Fox, B. (Ed.). (1988). *Family bonds and gender divisions: Readings in the sociology of the family.* Toronto: Canadian Scholars' Press.

Freidson, E. (1970). *Profession of medicine: A study of the sociology of applied knowledge.* New York: Dodd, Mead.

Freidson, E. (1989). The reorganization of the medical profession. In E. Freidson (Ed.), *Medical work in America: Essays on health care* (pp. 178-205). New Haven, CT: Yale University Press.

Friedland, R. B., & Summer, L. (1999). *Demography is not destiny.* Washington, DC: Gerontological Society of America, National Academy on an Aging Society.

Friedlander, D., & Burtless, G. (1995). *Five years after: Long-term effects of welfare-to-work programs.* New York: Russell Sage.

Fries, J. F. (1980). Aging, natural death, and the compression of morbidity. *New England Journal of Medicine, 303*(3), 130-135.

Fritz, M. (1990, January 8). Health. *Forbes,* pp. 180-182.

Fruedenheim, M. (1999, January 13). Concern rising about mergers in health plans. *New York Times,* pp. A1(L).

Fubini, S., & Stephanie, L. (1997, September/October). The ties that bind. *Health Systems Review,* 44-47.

Fuchs, V. R. (1988). The "competition revolution" in health care. *Health Affairs, 7*(3), 5-24.

Gallagher, L. (1999, January 11). The big money is in small towns. *Forbes,* pp. 182-183.

Geanaloplos, J., Mitchell, O.S., & Zeldes, S.P. (1999, May). "Would a Privatized Social Security System Really Pay a Higher Rate of Return?" Paper presented at the First Annual Joint Conference for the Retirement Research Consortium, "New Developments in Retirement Research," Washington, DC.

Geiger, H. J. (1981). Health policy, social policy, and the health of the aging: Prelude to a decade of disaster. In P. R. Lee, N. Ramsey, & I. Red (Eds.), *The nation's health* (pp. 389-394). San Francisco: Boyd & Fraser.

General Accounting Office. (1998). *Long-term care: Baby boom generation presents financing challenges* (Testimony of William Scanlon GAO/T-HEHS-98-107). Washington, DC: U.S. Senate Special Committee on Aging.

George, L. K. (1990). Social structure, social processes, and social psychological states. In R. H. Binstock & L. K. George (Eds.), *Handbook of aging and the social sciences* (pp. 186-200). San Diego, CA: Academic Press.

George, L. K. (1993). Sociological perspectives on life transitions. *Annual Review of Sociology, 19,* 353-373.

Gerstel, N., & Gallagher, S. (1994). Caring for kith and kin: Gender, employment, and the privatization of care. *Social Problems, 41,* 519-539.

Giddens, A. (1984). *The constitution of society: Outline of the theory of structuration.* Berkeley: University of California Press.

Giddens, A. (1990). *Capitalism and modern social theory: An analysis of the writings of Marx, Durkheim, and Max Weber.* Cambridge, UK: Cambridge University Press.

Giddens, A. (1991). *Modernity and self-identity: Self and society in the late modern age.* Cambridge, UK: Polity Press, in association with B. Blackwell, Oxford.

Giddens, A., & Held, D. (Eds.). (1982). *Classes, power and conflict: Classical and contemporary debates.* Berkeley: University of California Press.

Ginn, J., & Arber, S. (1995). Only connect: Gender relations and aging. In S. Arber & J. Ginn (Eds.), *Connecting gender and ageing: A sociological approach* (pp. 1-13). Philadelphia: Open University Press.

Ginzberg, E. (1988). For profit medicine: A reassessment. *New England Journal of Medicine, 319,* 757-761.

Gokhale, J., & Kotlikoff, L. J. (1999). Generational justice and generational accounting. In J. B. Williamson, D. M. Watts-Roy, & E. Kingson (Eds.), *The generational equity debate* (pp. 75-86). New York: Columbia University Press.

Gold, D. A., Lo, C. Y. H., & Wright, E. O. (1975). Recent developments in Marxist theories of the capitalist state. *Monthly Review: An Independent Socialist Magazine, 27*(5), 29-43.

Gornick, M. E., Eggers, P. W., Reilly, T. W., Mentnech, R. M., Fitterman, L. K., Kucken, L. E., & Vladeck, B. C. (1996). Effects of race and income on mortality and use of services among Medicare beneficiaries. *New England Journal of Medicine, 335*(11), 791-799.

Gouldner, A. W. (1970). *The coming crisis of Western sociology.* New York: Basic Books.

Gouldner, A. W. (1973). *For sociology: Renewal and critique in sociology today.* New York: Basic Books.

Grad, S. (1998). *Income of the aged chartbook, 1996.* Washington, DC: Social Security Administration.

Graebner, W. (1980). *A history of retirement: The meaning and function of an American institution, 1885-1978.* New Haven, CT: Yale University Press.

Gramsci, A., Hoare, Q., & Nowell-Smith, G. (1971). *Selections from the prison notebooks of Antonio Gramsci.* London: Lawrence & Wishart.

Gray, B. H. (1986). *For-profit enterprise in health care.* Washington, DC: National Academy Press.

Green, L. W., Kreuter, M. W., Deeds, S. G., & Partridge, K. B. (1980). *Health education planning: A diagnostic approach.* Palo Alto, CA: Mayfield.

Gronbjerg, J. (1987). Patterns of institutional relations in the welfare state: Public mandates and the nonprofit sector. In S. A. Ostrander & S. Langton (Eds.), *Shifting the debate: Public/private sector relations in the modern welfare state* (pp. 64-80). New Brunswick, NJ: Transaction Books.

Gruenberg, E. M. (1977). The failures of success. *Milbank Memorial Fund Quarterly/Health and Society, 55*(1), 3-24.

Gubrium, J. F. (1967). *The myth of the golden years: A socio-environmental theory of aging.* Springfield, IL: Charles C Thomas.

Gubrium, J. F., & Holstein, J. A. (1999). Constructionist perspectives on aging. In V. L. Bengtson & K. W. Schaie (Eds.), *Handbook of theories of aging* (pp. 287-305). New York: Springer.

Gueron, J., Pauley, E., & Lougy, C. (1991). *From welfare to work.* New York: Russell Sage.

Guillemard, A. M. (1980). *La vielless l'etat.* Paris: Presses Universitaires de France.

Guillemard, A. M. (1993). Older workers and the labour market. In A. Walker, J. Alber, & A. M. Guillemard (Eds.), *Older people in Europe: Social and economic policies* (pp. 35-51). Brussels: Commission on the European Communities.

Guralnik, J. M., & Simonsick, E. M. (1993). Physical disability in older Americans. *Journal of Gerontology, 48*, 3-10.

Gurr, T. R. (1970). *Why men rebel.* Princeton, NJ: Princeton University Press.

Haan, M., Kaplan, G., & Syme, S. (1989). Old observations and new thoughts. In J. Bunker, D. Gomby, & B. Kehrer (Eds.), *Pathways to health: The role of social factors* (pp. 76-117). Menlo Park, CA: Henry J. Kaiser Family Foundation.

Haan, M., Kaplan, G. A., & Camacho, T. (1987). Poverty and health. Prospective evidence from the Alameda County Study. *American Journal of Epidemiology, 125*(6), 989-998.

Habermas, J. (1962). *Strukturwandel der eOffentlichkeit: Untersuchungen zu einer Kategorie der beurgerlichen Gesellschaft.* Neuwied, Berlin: Luchterhand.

Habermas, J. (1970). *Toward a rational society: Student protest, science, and politics.* Boston: Beacon.

Habermas, J. (1971). *Knowledge and human interests.* Boston: Beacon.

Habermas, J. (1973). *Theory and practice.* Boston: Beacon.

Habermas, J. (1975). *Legitimation crisis.* Boston: Beacon.

Habermas, J. (1984). What does a legitimation crisis mean today? Legitimation problems in late capitalism. In W. E. Connolly (Ed.), *Legitimacy and the state* (pp. 134-155). New York: New York University Press.

Hagestad, G. O. (1990). Social perspectives on the life course. In R. H. Binstock & L. K. George (Eds.), *Handbook of aging and the social sciences* (pp. 151-168). San Diego, CA: Academic Press.

Hahn, M., & Kaplan, G. A. (1985). The contribution of socioeconomic position to minority health. In M. Heckler (Ed.), *Report of the Secretary's Task Force on Black and Minority Health.* Washington, DC: U.S. Department of Health and Human Services.

Hall, M., & Sangl, J. (1987, October). *Impact of Medicare's PPS on long-term care providers.* Paper presented at the annual meeting of the American Public Health Association.

Hall, P. (1987). Abandoning the rhetoric of independence: Reflections on the nonprofit sector in the post-liberal era. In S. A. Ostrander & S. Langton (Eds.), *Shifting the debate: Public/private sector relations in the modern welfare state* (pp. 11-28). New Brunswick, NJ: Transaction Books.

Hall, S. (1996). Gramsci's relevance for the study of race and ethnicity. In D. Morley & K.-H. Clan (Eds.), *Stuart Hall: Critical dialogues in cultural studies* (pp. 411-440). New York: Routledge.

Hamilton, G., & Brock, T. (1994). *The JOBS evaluation: Early lessons from seven sites.* New York: Russell Sage.

Hansmann, H. B. (1980). The role of nonprofit enterprise. *Yale Law Journal, 89,* 835-901.

Harding, S. (1996). Standpoint epistemology (a feminist version): How social disadvantage creates epistemic advantage. In S. P. Turner (Ed.), *Social theory and sociology: The classics and beyond* (pp. 146-160). Cambridge, MA: Basil Blackwell.

Harrington, C. (1996). The nursing home industry: Public policy in the 1990s. In P. Brown (Ed.), *Perspectives in medical sociology,* 2nd ed. (pp. 515-534). Prospect Heights, IL: Waveland.

Harrington, C. (1999). The nursing home industry: The failure of reform efforts. In M. Minkler & C. L. Estes (Eds.), *Critical gerontology: Perspectives from political and moral economy* (pp. 221-232). Amityville, NY: Baywood.

Harrington, C., Carrillo, H., Thollaug, S., & Summers, P. (1999). *Nursing facilities, staffing, residents, and facility deficiencies, 1991-1997.* San Francisco: University of California.

Harrington, C., Cassel, C., Estes, C. L., Woolhandler, S., & Himmelstein, D. V. (1991). A national long-term care program for the United States: A caring vision (Working Group on Long-Term Care Program Design, Physicians for a National Health Program). *Journal of the American Medical Association, 266*(21), 3023-3029.

Harrington, C., Swan, J. H., Griffin, C., Clemena, W., Bedney, B., Carrillo, H. M., & Shostak, S. (1998). *1996 state data book on long term care programs and market characteristics.* San Francisco: University of California.

Harrington Meyer, M. (1990). Family status and poverty among older women: The gendered distribution of retirement income in the U.S. *Social Problems, 37*(4), 551-563.

Harrington Meyer, M. (1996). Making claims as workers or wives: The distribution of Social Security benefits. *American Sociological Review, 61*(3), 449-465.

Hart, P. D., & associates. (1990). *Report of poll results on long term care.* Washington, DC: Families USA Foundation.

Hartmann, H. (1981). The unhappy marriage of Marxism and feminism. In L. Sargent (Ed.), *Women and revolution: A discussion of the unhappy marriage of Marxism and feminism* (pp. 1-41). Boston: South End.

Hayes, J. (1998, January 12). Health care services (Annual report on American industry). *Forbes,* pp. 180-181.

Health Care Financing Administration. (1998a). *National health expenditures aggregate and per capita amounts, percent distribution and average annual percent growth, by source of funds: Selected calendar years 1960-1998.* Health Care Financing Administration, Office of the Actuary: National Health Statistics Group. Retrieved May 15, 2000, from the World Wide Web: www.hcfa.gov/stats/nhe-oact/tables/t1.htm

Health Care Financing Administration. (1998b). *National health expenditures and selected economic indicators, levels and average annual percent change: Selected calendar years 1970-2008.* Health Care Financing Administration, Office of the Actuary: National

Health Statistics Group. Retrieved May 15, 2000, from the World Wide Web: www.hcfa.gov/stats/nhe-proj/proj1998/tables/table1.htm

Held, D., & Thompson, J. B. (1982). *Habermas: Critical debates.* Cambridge: MIT Press.

Hendricks, J. (1992). Generations and the generation of theory in social gerontology. *International Journal of Aging and Human Development, 35*(1), 31-47.

Hendricks, J., & Leedham, C. (1991). Dependency or empowerment? Toward a moral and political economy of aging. In M. Minkler & C. L. Estes (Eds.), *Critical perspectives on aging: The political and moral economy of growing old* (pp. 51-66). Amityville, NY: Baywood.

Henretta, J. C., & Campbell, R. T. (1976). Status attainment and status maintenance: A study of stratification in old age. *American Sociological Review, 41*(6), 981-992.

Henwood, D. (1999, May/June). TV on Social Security: It's broke, fix it. *EXTRA!* pp. 8-12.

Hernes, H. M. (1987). *Welfare state and woman power: Essays in state feminism.* Oslo: Norwegian University Press.

Herzog, A. R., Kahn, R. L., Morgan, J. N., Jackson, J. S., & Antonucci, T. C. (1989). Age differences in productive activities. *Journal of Gerontology, 44*(4), S129-S138.

Himmelstein, D. U., & Woolhandler, S. (1986). Cost without benefit: Administrative waste in the U.S. *New England Journal of Medicine, 314,* 440-441.

Himmelweit, S. (1983). Reproduction. In T. Bottomore (Ed.), *Dictionary of Marxist thought* (pp. 417-419). Cambridge, MA: Harvard University Press.

Hodgkinson, V. A. (1996). *Nonprofit almanac 1996-1997: Dimensions of the independent sector.* San Francisco: Jossey-Bass.

Hodgkinson, V. A., & Weitzman, M. S. (1984). *Dimensions of the independent sector: A statistical profile.* Washington, DC: Independent Sector.

Hoffman, C., & Rice, D. (1996). *Chronic illness.* Princeton, NJ: Robert Wood Johnson Foundation.

Holstein, M. (1992). Productive aging: A feminist critique. *Journal of Aging and Social Policy, 4*(3-4), 17-34.

Holstein, M. (1999). Women and productive aging: Troubling implications. In M. Minkler & C. L. Estes (Eds.), *Critical gerontology: Perspectives from political and moral economy* (pp. 359-373). Amityville, NY: Baywood.

House, J. S., Landis, K. R., & Umberson, D. (1994). Social relationships and health. In P. Conrad & R. Kern (Eds.), *The sociology of health and illness: Critical perspectives* (4th ed., pp. 83-92). New York: St. Martin's.

House, J. S., Kessler, R. C., & Herzog, A. R. (1990). Age, socioeconomic status, and health. *Milbank Quarterly, 68*(3), 383-411.

Howe, R. (1999, February 6). The People vs. HMOs. *Time,* pp. 46-47.

Iglehart, J. K. (1982). Health care and American business. *New England Journal of Medicine, 306*(2), 120-124.

Iglehart, J. K. (1989). The debate over physician ownership of health care facilities. *New England Journal of Medicine, 321,* 198-204.

Illich, I. (1976). *Medical nemesis: The expropriation of health.* New York: Pantheon.

Independent Sector. (1995). *Giving and volunteering in the United States: Vol. II.* Washington, DC: Author.

Independent Sector. (1988). *The taxation of nonprofits: A state by state summary.* Washington, DC: Author.

InterStudy. (1989). *Findings on open-ended HMOs reports by InterStudy* [Press release]. Excelsior, MD: Author.

Isaacson, E. (1993, April 14). Prescription for change. *San Francisco Bay Guardian.*

Jacobs, L., & Shapiro, R. (1994). *The news media's coverage of Social Security: 1977-1994.* Unpublished report to National Academy of Social Insurance, Washington, DC.

Jaggar, A. M., & Rothenberg, P. S. (1984). *Feminist frameworks.* New York: McGraw-Hill.

Jaspen, B. (1999, January 31). AMA firing impolitic—or just politics? *Chicago Tribune,* p. 5.

Jette, A. M. (1996). Disability trends and transitions. In R. H. Binstock & L. K. George (Eds.), *Handbook of aging and the social sciences* (4th ed., pp. 94-116). San Diego, CA: Academic Press.

Jones, K. (1990). Citizenship in a woman friendly polity. *Signs, 15*(4), 781-812.

Jones, V. Y., & Estes, C. L. (1997). Older women: Income, retirement, and health. In S. B. Ruzek, V. L. Olesen, & A. E. Clarke (Eds.), *Women's health: Complexities and differences* (pp. 425-445). Columbus: Ohio State University Press.

Kagarlitsky, B. (1999). The challenge for the Left: Reclaiming the state. In L. Panitch & C. Leys (Eds.), *Social Register 1999: Global capitalism versus democracy* (pp. 294-313). New York: Monthly Review Press.

Kane, R. L. (1999). Examining the efficiency of home care. *Journal of Aging, 11,* 322-340.

Kaplan, G., & Haan, M. (1989). Is there a role for prevention among the elderly? Epidemiological evidence from the Alameda County Study. In K. Bond & M. G. Ory (Eds.), *Aging and health care: Social science and policy perspectives* (pp. 27-51). New York: Routledge.

Kapp, M. B. (1995). Legal and ethical issues in family caregiving and the role of public policy. In R. A. Kane & J. D. Penrod (Eds.), *Family caregiving in an aging society* (pp. 123-143). Thousand Oaks, CA: Sage.

Kassirer, J. (1997). Mergers and acquisitions: Who benefits? Who loses? *New England Journal of Medicine, 334,* 722-723.

Kempler, P. (1992). The use of formal and informal home care by the disabled elderly. *Health Services Research, 27,* 421-451.

Kimbrell, A. (Ed.). (1996). *Biocolonization: The patenting of life and the global market in body parts.* San Francisco: Sierra Club Books.

King, G. (1996). Institutional racism and the medical/health complex: A conceptual analysis. *Ethnicity and Disease, 6*(1-2), 30-46.

Kingson, E., & Williamson, J. B. (1999). Why privatizing Social Security is a bad idea. In J. B. Williamson, D. M. Watts-Roy, & E. Kingson (Eds.), *The generational equity debate* (pp. 204-219). New York: Columbia University Press.

Knuttila, M. (1996). *Introducing sociology: A critical perspective.* New York: Oxford University Press.

Kohli, M. (1987). Retirement and the moral economy: An historical interpretation of the German case. *Journal of Aging Studies, 1,* 125-144.

Kohli, M. (1988). Aging as a challenge for sociological theory. *Ageing and Society, 8,* 367-394.

Kohli, M., Guillemard, A. M., & Gunsteren, H. V. (Eds.). (1991). *Time for retirement: Comparative studies of early exit from the labor force.* Cambridge, MA: Cambridge University Press.

Komisar, H., Lambrew, J., & Feder, J. (1996). *Long-term care for the elderly.* New York: Commonwealth Fund.

Kramarae, C., & Treichler, P. A. (1992). *Amazons, bluestockings and crones: A feminist dictionary.* London: Pandora.

Kramer, M. (1980). The rising pandemic of mental disorders and associated chronic diseases and disabilities. *Acta Psychiatrica Scandinavica, 62*(285, Suppl.), 382-397.

Kramer, R. (1987). Voluntary agencies and the personal social services. In W. W. Powell (Ed.), *The nonprofit sector: A research handbook* (pp. 240-276). New Haven, CT: Yale University Press.

Krause, E. A. (1996). *Death of the guilds: Professions, states, and the advance of capitalism, 1930 to the present.* New Haven, CT: Yale University Press.

Krieger, N., & Fee, E. (1994). Social class: The missing link in the U.S. health data. *Journal of Health Services, 24,* 25-44.

Krieger, N., Rowley, D. L., Herman, A. A., Avery, B., & Phillips, M. T. (1993). Racism, sexism, and social class: Implications for studies of health, disease, and well-being. *American Journal of Preventive Medicine, 9*(6, Suppl), 82-122.

Krieger, N., Williams, D. R., & Moss, N. E. (1997). Measuring social class in U.S. public health research: Concepts, methodologies, and guidelines. *Annual Review of Public Health, 18,* 341-378.

Krivo, L. J., & Peterson, R. D. (1996). Extremely disadvantaged neighborhoods and urban crime. *Social Forces, 75,* 619-648.

Kuttner, R. (1999). The American health care system: Health insurance coverage. *New England Journal of Medicine, 340,* 163-168.

Lane, R. (1986). Market justice, political justice. *American Political Science, 80,* 383-402.

Lantz, P. M., House, J. S., Lepkowski, J. M., Williams, D. R., Mero, R. P., & Chen, J. (1998). Socioeconomic factors, health behaviors, and mortality: Results from a nationally representative prospective study of U.S. adults. *Journal of the American Medical Association, 279*(21), 1703-1708.

LaPlante, M. P., & Carlson, D. (1996). *Disability in the U.S.: Prevalence and causes, disability statistics* (Report No. 7). Washington, DC: U.S. Department of Education, National Institute on Disability and Rehabilitation Research.

LaPlante, M. P. (1991). *Disability risks of chronic illnesses and impairments* [microfilm]. Washington, DC: U.S. Department of Education, Office of Special Education and Rehabilitative Services, National Institute on Disability and Rehabilitation Research.

Larrañaga, O. (1999). Health sector reforms in Chile. In G. Perr & D. Leipziger (Eds.), *Chile: Recent policy lessons and emerging challenges* (pp. 189-225). Washington, DC: World Bank.

Lasch, C. (1978). *The culture of narcissism: American life in an age of diminishing expectations.* New York: Norton.

Lee, P. R. (1984). Health policy and the health of the public: A two-hundred year perspective. *Mobius, 4*(3), 95-113.

Lee, P. R. (2000). Introduction to Chapter 1. In P. R. Lee & C. L. Estes (Eds.), *The nation's health* (6th ed., p. 5). Boston: Jones & Bartlett.

Lee, P. R., & Etheredge, L. (1989). Clinical freedom: Two lessons for the U.K. from U.S. experience with privatisation of health care. *Lancet, 1*(8632), 263-265.

LeGrand, J. (1987, November). *The privatization of welfare.* Paper presented at the National Conference on Public Expenditure, Dublin, Ireland: Institute of Public Administration.

Lerner, G. (1986). *The creation of patriarchy.* New York: Oxford University Press.

LeRoy, L. (1979). *The political economy of U.S. federal health policy: A closer look at Medicare.* Unpublished manuscript, University of California, San Francisco.

Levine, C. (1999). Home sweet hospital: The nature and limits of private responsibilities for home health care. *Journal of Aging Studies, 11,* 341-359.

Levitas, R. (1986). Competition and compliance: The utopias of the new right. In R. Levitas (Ed.), *The ideology of the new right* (pp. 80-106). Cambridge, MA: Polity.

Leys, C. (1999). The public sphere and the media: Market supremacy versus democracy. In L. Panitch & C. Leys (Eds.), *Social Register 1999: Global capitalism versus democracy* (pp. 314-335). New York: Monthly Review.

Lipset, S. M. (1960). *Political man: The social bases of politics.* Garden City, NY: Doubleday.

Lowenthal, M., & Robinson, B. (1976). Social networks and isolation. In R. H. Binstock & E. Shanas (Eds.), *Handbook of aging and the social sciences* (pp. 432-456). New York: Van Nostrand Reinhold.

Lowenthal, M. F. (1975). Psychosocial variations across the adult life course: Frontiers for research and policy. *The Gerontologist, 15*(Pt 1), 6-12.

Lynch, M., & Estes, C. L. (1997). Is managed care good for older persons? In A. E. Scharlach & L. W. Kaye (Eds.), *Controversial issues in aging* (pp. 120-123). Boston: Allyn & Bacon.

Lynch, M., & Minkler, M. (1999). Impacts of proposed restructuring of Medicare and Medicaid on the elderly: A conceptual framework and analysis. In M. Minkler & C. L. Estes (Eds.), *Critical gerontology: Perspectives from political and moral economy* (pp. 185-201). Amityville, NY: Baywood.

MacKinnon, C. A. (1982). Feminism, Marxism, method, and the state: An agenda for theory. *Signs, 7*(3), 515-544.

MacKinnon, C. A. (1989). *Toward a feminist theory of the state.* Cambridge, MA: Harvard University Press.

Manning, N. P. (1985). *Social problems and welfare ideology.* Brookfield, VT: Gower.

Manton, K. G., Corder, L., & Stallard, E. (1997). Chronic disability trends in elderly in United States populations: 1982-1994. *Proceedings of the National Academy of Sciences of the USA, 94,*(6), 2593-2598.

Manton, K. G. (1982). Changing concepts of morbidity and mortality in the elderly population. *Health and Society, 60*(2), 183-244.

Manton, K. G., Corder, L. S., & Stallard, E. (1993). Changes in the use of personal assistance and special equipment from 1982 to 1989: Results from the 1982 and 1989 NLTCS. *The Gerontologist, 33,* 168-176.

Manton, K. G., Singer, B. H., & Suzman, R. (1993). *Forecasting the health of elderly populations.* New York: Springer-Verlag.

Manton, K. G., Stallard, E., & Wing, S. (1991). Analyses of black and white differentials in the age trajectory of mortality in two closed cohort studies. *Statistics in Medicine, 10*(7), 1043-1059.

Marmor, T., Cook, F. L., & Scher, S. (1999). Social Security and the politics of generational conflict. In J. B. Williamson, D. M. Watts-Roy, & E. Kingson (Eds.), *The generational equity debate* (pp. 185-203). New York: Columbia University Press.

Marmor, T., Schlesinger, M., & Smithey, R. (1987). Non-profit organizations and health care. In W. W. Powell (Ed.), *The nonprofit sector: a research handbook* (pp. 221-239). New Haven, CT: Yale University Press.

Marmor, T. R., Mashaw, J. L., & Harvey, P. (1990). *America's misunderstood welfare state: Persistent myths, enduring realities.* New York: Basic Books.

Marmot, M., Kogevinas, M., & Elston, M. (1987). Social/economic status and disease. *Annual Review of Public Health, 8,* 111-135.

Marshall, V. W. (1999). Analyzing social theories of aging. In V. L. Bengston & K. W. Schaie (Ed.), *Handbook of theories of aging* (pp. 434-455). New York: Springer.

Marshall, V. W. (1996). The state of theory in aging and the social sciences. In R. H. E. Binstock, L. K. George, V. W. Marshall, G. C. Myers, & J. H. Schulz (Eds.), *Handbook of aging and the social sciences* (4th ed.) (pp. 12-30). San Diego: Academic Press.

Marshall, V. W., & Tindale, J. A. (1978). Notes for a radical gerontology. *International Journal of Aging and Human Development, 9*(2), 163-175.

Marsteller, J., Bovbjerg, R., & Nichols, L. (1998). Nonprofit conversion: Theory, evidence, and state policy options. *Health Services Research, 33,* 5.

Marx, K. (1978). Capital. In R. F. Tucker (Ed.), *Capital* (2nd ed., Vol. 1). New York: Norton. (Original work published 1887)

McGinnis, J. M., & Foege, W. H. (1993). Actual causes of death in the United States. *Journal of the American Medical Association, 270*(18), 2207-2212.

McKenzie, K. (1998). Toward a comprehensive model for the impact of racism on the health of African-Americans [abstract]. *Abstract Book/Association for Health Services Research, 15,* 335.

McKeown, T. (1978). Determinants of health. *Human Nature, 1*(4), 60-67.

McKeown, T. (1997). Determinants of health. In P. R. Lee, C. L. Estes, & L. Close (Eds.), *The nation's health* (pp. 9-17). Boston, MA: Jones & Bartlett.

McKinlay, J. B. (1985). *Issues in the political economy of health care.* New York: Tavistock.

McKinlay, J. B., & Hafferty, F. W. (1993). *The changing medical profession: An international perspective.* New York: Oxford University Press.

McKinlay, J. B., & McKinlay, S. M. (1977). The questionable contribution of medical measures to the decline of mortality in the United States in the twentieth century. *Milbank Memorial Fund Quarterly/Health and Society, 55,* 405-428.

McKinlay, J. B., McKinlay, S. M., & Beaglehole, R. (1989). Trends in death and disease and the contribution of medical measures. In H. E. Freeman & S. Levine (Eds.), *Handbook of medical sociology* (pp. 14-45). Englewood Cliffs, NJ: Prentice Hall.

McKinlay, J. B., & Stoeckle, J. D. (1988). Corporatization and the social transformation of doctoring. *International Journal of Health Services, 18*(2), 191-205.

McKinlay, J. B., & Stoeckle, J. D. (1994). Corporatization and the social transformation of doctoring. In P. Conrad & R. Kern (Eds.), *The sociology of health and illness: Critical perspectives* (pp. 182-193). New York: St. Martin's.

McMullin, J. A. (1995). Theorizing age and gender relations: In S. Arber & J. Ginn (Eds.), *Connecting gender and ageing: A sociological approach* (pp. 30-41). Philadelphia, PA: Open University Press.

McNamee, M. (1997, March 17). Health-care inflation: It's baaack! *Business Week*, pp. 28-30.

Mechanic, D. (1983). *Handbook of health, health care, and the health professions.* New York: Free Press.

Medpac. (1999). *Selected Medicare issues* (Report to Congress). Washington, DC: Medicare Payment Advisory Commission.

Melendez, S. E. (1999, October). *The state of the sector, an address by Sara E. Melendez President & CEO, Independent Sector.* Paper presented at the Independent Sector Annual Conference, Los Angeles, CA.

Merelman, R. M. (1966). Learning and legitimacy. *American Political Science Review, 60*(3), 548.

Minkler, M., & Cole, T. (1999). Political and moral economy: Getting to know one another. In M. Minkler & C. L. Estes (Eds.), *Critical gerontology: Perspectives from political and moral economy* (pp. 37-49). Amityville, NY: Baywood.

Minkler, M., & Cole, T. R. (1991). Political and moral economy: Not such strange bedfellows. In M. Minkler & C. L. Estes (Eds.), *Critical perspectives on aging: The political and moral economy of growing old* (pp. 37-49). Amityville, NY: Baywood.

Minkler, M., & Estes, C. L. (Eds.). (1984). *Readings in the political economy of aging.* Farmingdale, NY: Baywood.

Minkler, M., & Estes, C. L. (Eds.). (1991). *Critical perspectives on aging: The political and moral economy of growing old.* Amityville, NY: Baywood.

Minkler, M., & Estes, C. L. (Eds.). (1999). *Critical gerontology: Perspectives from political and moral economy.* Amityville, NY: Baywood.

Minkler, M., & Fullarton, J. E. (1981, November-December). *Health promotion, health maintenance, and disease prevention for the elderly.* Paper presented at the 1981 White House Conference on Aging, Washington, DC.

Mitchell, J. (1966). *Women: The longest revolution.* Boston, MA: New England Free Press.

Moen, P., Robison, J., & Fields, V. (1994). Women's work and caregiving roles: A life course approach. *Journal of Gerontology, 49,* S176-S186.

Mollica, R. L., & Riley, T. (1997). *Managed care for low income elders dually eligible for Medicaid and Medicare: A snapshot of state and federal activity.* Portland, ME: National Academy for State Health Policy.

Montgomery, R. V. (1999). The family role in the context of long-term care. *Journal of Aging Studies, 11,* 383-416.

Moody, H. R. (1988a). *Abundance of life: Human development policies for an aging society.* New York: Columbia University Press.

Moody, H. R. (1988b). Toward a critical gerontology: The contributions of the humanities to theories of aging. In J. E. Birren, V. L. Bengtson, & D. E. Deutchman (Eds.), *Emergent theories of aging* (pp. 19-40). New York: Springer.

Moody, H. R. (1993a). Age, productivity, and transcendence. In S. A. Bass, F. G. Caro, & Y. P. Chen (Eds.), *Achieving a productive aging society* (pp. 28-40). Westport, CT: Auburn House.

Moody, H. R. (1993b). Overview: What is critical gerontology and why is it important. In T. R. Cole (Ed.), *Voices and visions of aging: Toward a critical gerontology* (pp. xv-xxi). New York: Springer.

Moody, H. R. (1997). *The five stages of the soul.* New York: Doubleday.

Moody, H. R. (1998). *Aging: Concepts and controversies* (2nd ed.). Thousand Oaks, CA: Pine Forge.

Moon, M., & Gage, B. (1997). *Key Medicare provisions in the Balanced Budget Act of 1997* (The Public Policy and Aging Report). Washington, DC: National Academy on Aging and the Gerontological Society of America.

Morgan, J. (1988). The relationship of housing and living arrangements to the productivity of older people. In Committee on an Aging Society (Ed.), *The social and built environment in an older society* (pp. 250-280). Washington, DC: National Academy Press.

Morioka-Douglas, N., & Yeo, G. (1990). *Aging and health: Asian/Pacific Island elders* (Working Paper No. 3, ethnogeriatric review). Stanford, CA: Stanford Geriatric Education Center.

Munnell, A. H. (1999). America can afford to grow old. In J. B. Williamson, D. M. Watts-Roy, & E. Kingson (Eds.), *The generational equity debate* (pp. 117-139). New York: Columbia University Press.

Munnichs, J. M. A., & van den Heuvel, W. J. A. (Eds.). (1976). *Dependency or interdependency in old age.* The Hague, Netherlands: Martinus Nijhoff.

Myles, J. (1984). *Old age in the welfare state: The political economy of public pensions.* Boston, MA: Little, Brown.

Myles, J. (1991). Postwar capitalism and the extension of Social Security into a retirement wage. In M. Minkler & C. L. Estes (Eds.), *Critical perspectives on aging: The political and moral economy of growing old* (pp. 293-309). Amityville, NY: Baywood.

Myles, J., & Quadagno, J. S. (1991). *States, labor markets, and the future of old age policy.* Philadelphia, PA: Temple University Press.

Myles, J. F. (1982). Population aging and the elderly. In D. Forcese & S. Richer (Eds.), *Social issues: Sociological views of Canada.* Ontario, Canada: Prentice Hall.

Myles, J. F. (1996). When markets fail: Social welfare in Canada and the United States. In G. Esping-Andersen (Ed.), *Welfare states in transition: National adaptations in global economies* (pp. 116-140). London: Sage.

National Association for Home Care. (1993). *Basic statistics about home care—1993* (Report). Washington, DC: Author.

National Academy of Social Insurance. (1994). *When support and confidence are at odds: The public's understanding of the Social Security program.* Washington, DC: Author.

National Bipartisan Commission on the Future of Medicare. (1999, March 16). *Building a better Medicare for today and tomorrow.* Retrieved in May 2000 from the World Wide Web: thomas.loc.gov/medicare/bbmtt31599.html

National Center for Health Statistics. (1993). *Health data on older Americans: United States, 1992* (Vital and Health Statistics, Series 3: Analytic and Epidemiological Studies 27). Washington, DC: Author.

National Center for Health Statistics. (1994). *The 1992 National Health Interview Survey.* Washington, DC: Author.

National Center for Health Statistics. (1995). *The 1995 National Health Interview Survey.* Washington, DC: Author.

National Center for Health Statistics. (1998). *Health, United States, 1998 with socioeconomic status and health chartbook.* Hyattsville, MD: Author.(DDHS Pub. No. PHS 98-1232)

National Center for Health Statistics. (1999a). *Current estimates from the National Health Interview Survey, 1996* (Series 10, DHHS Publication No. PHS 99-1528). Washington, DC: Author.

National Center for Health Statistics. (1999b). *Health, United States, 1999 with health and aging chartbook* (DHHS Publication No. 99-1232). Washington, DC: National Center for Health Statistics.

National Economic Council. (1998, October). *Women and retirement security.* Paper presented at the Interagency Working Group on Social Security, Washington, DC.

Navarro, V. (1976). *Medicine under capitalism.* New York: Prodist.

Navarro, V. (1982). The labor process and health: A historical materialist interpretation. *International Journal of Health Services, 12,* 5-29.

Navarro, V. (1984). Political economy of government cuts for the elderly. In M. Minkler & C. L. Estes (Eds.), *Readings in the political economy of aging* (pp. 37-46). Farmingdale, NY: Baywood.

Navarro, V. (1986). *Crisis, health, and medicine: A social critique.* New York: Tavistock.

Navarro, V. (1990). Race or class versus race and class: Mortality differentials in the United States. *Lancet, 336,* 1238-1240.

Navarro, V. (1995). Why Congress did not enact health care reform. *Journal of Health Politics, Policy and Law, 20,* 455-461.

Navarro, V., & Berman, D. M. (1983). *Health and work under capitalism: An international perspective.* Farmingdale, NY: Baywood.

NBC News/*Wall Street Journal* Poll. (1998). *Election issues: Poll, June 18-21, 1998.* Retrieved July 9, 1998, from PollingReport.com on the World Wide Web: pollingreport.com/issues.htm

NBC News/*Wall Street Journal* Poll. (1999). *Election issues: Poll, December 9-12, 1999.* Retrieved February 22, 2000, from PollingReport.com on the World Wide Web: pollingreport.com/prioriti.htm

Nelson, G. (1982). Social class and public policy for the elderly. *Social Service Review, 56*(1), 85-107.

Nelson, J. I. (1995). *Post-industrial capitalism: Exploring economic inequality in America.* Thousand Oaks, CA: Sage.

Neugarten, B. L. (1964). *Personality in middle and late life: Empirical studies.* New York: Atherton.

Neugarten, B. L., Havinghurst, R. J., & Tobin, S. S. (1968). Personality and patterns of aging. In B. L. Neugarten (Ed.), *Middle age and aging: A reader in social psychology.* Chicago: University of Chicago Press.

Newcomer, R. J., Yordi, C., DuNah, R., Fox, P., & Wilkinson, A. (1999). Effects of the Medicare Alzheimer's Disease Demonstration on caregiver burden and depression. *Health Services Research, 34*(3), 669-689.

Not-for-profits prepare to battle local tax assessor. (1987). *AHA News, 23*(16), 5.

O'Connor, J. (1973). *The fiscal crisis of the state.* New York: St. Martin's.

O'Connor, J. (1984). *Accumulation crisis.* New York: Basil Blackwell.

O'Connor, J. (1987). *The meaning of crisis: A theoretical introduction.* New York: Basil Blackwell.

O'Connor, J. (1993a). Gender, class, citizenship in the comparative analysis of welfare state regimes: Theoretical & methodological issues. *British Journal of Sociology, 44,* 501-518.

O'Connor, J. S. (1993b). *Understanding women in welfare states* (Report funded by SSHRC grant). Hamilton, Ontario: McMaster University.

O'Connor, J. S., Orloff, A. S., & Shaver, S. (1999). *States, markets, families: Gender, liberalism and social policy in Australia, Canada, Great Britain and the United States.* Cambridge, UK: Cambridge University Press.

Offe, C. (1973). *The abolition of market control and the problems of legitimacy.* Working Papers on the Kapitalstate, I and II, Max Planck Institute, Saarbrücken, Germany.

Offe, C. (1976). Crisis of crisis management. *International Journal of Political Science, 6,* 29-67.

Offe, C., & Keane, J. (1984). *Contradictions of the welfare state.* Cambridge, MA: MIT Press.

Offe, C., & Ronge, V. (1982). Thesis on the theory of the state. In A. Giddens & D. Held (Eds.), *Classes, power, and conflict* (pp. 249-256). Berkeley: University of California Press.

Oliver, M. L., & Shapiro, T. M. (1995). *Black wealth/white wealth: A new perspective on racial inequality.* New York: Routledge.

Olshansky, S. J., Rudberg, M. A., Carnes, B. A., Cassel, C. K., & Brody, J. A. (1991). Trading off longer life for worsening health: The expansion of morbidity hypothesis. *Journal of Aging and Health, 3*(2), 194-216.

Olson, L. K. (1994). Women and Social Security: A progressive approach. *Journal of Aging and Social Policy, 6,* 43-56.

O'Rand, A. (1996). The cumulative stratification of the life course. In R. Binstock & L. George (Eds.), *Handbook of aging and the social sciences* (pp. 188-207). New York: Academic Press.

O'Rand, A., & National Academy on Aging. (1994). *The vulnerable majority: Older women in transition* (Advisory Panel Report). Syracuse, NY: Syracuse University.

Orloff, A. S. (1993). Gender and the social rights of citizenship: The comparative analysis of gender relations and welfare states. *American Sociological Review, 58*(3), 303-329.

Ostrander, S. A. (1987). Toward implications for research, theory, and policy on nonprofits and voluntarism. In S. A. Ostrander & S. Langton (Eds.), *Shifting the debate: Public/private sector relations in the modern welfare state* (pp. 126-133). New Brunswick, NJ: Transaction Books.

Ostrander, S. A., & Langton, S. (Eds.). (1987). *Shifting the debate: Public/private sector relations in the modern welfare state.* New Brunswick, NJ: Transaction Books.

Pampel, F. C. (1994). Population aging, class context, and age inequality in public spending. *American Journal of Sociology, 100*(1), 153-196.

Pampel, F. C. (1998). *Aging, social inequality, and public policy.* Thousand Oaks, CA: Pine Forge.

Pampel, F. C., & Williamson, J. (1995). Age structure, politics and cross national patterns of public pension expenditures. *American Sociological Review, 50,* 787-798.

Pampel, F. C., & Williamson, J. B. (1989). *Age, class, politics, and the welfare state.* New York: Cambridge University Press.

Pardes, H., Manton, K. G., Lander, E. S., Tolley, H. D., Ullian, A. D., & Palmer, H. (1999). Effects of medical research on health care and economy. *Science, 283*(5398), 36-37.

Parenti, M. (1999). Reflections on the politics of culture. *Monthly Review: An Independent Socialist Magazine, 50*(9), 11-18.

Parsons, T. (1951). *The social system.* Glencoe, IL: Free Press.

Pascall, G. (1986). *Social policy: A feminist analysis.* New York: Tavistock.

Pateman, C. (1989). *The disorder of women: Democracy, feminism, and political theory.* Stanford, CA: Stanford University Press.

Pear, R. (1997, October). Health insurers skirting new law, officials report. *New York Times,* p. AI.

Pearlin, L. I., Aneshensel, C. S., Mullan, J. T., & Whitlatch, C. J. (1996). Caregiving and its social support. In R. H. Binstock & L. K. George (Eds.), *Handbook of aging and the social sciences* (4th ed., pp. 283-302). San Diego, CA: Academic Press.

Pescosolido, B. A., & Kronenfeld, J. J. (1995). Health, illness, and healing in an uncertain era: Challenges from and for medical sociology. *Journal of Health and Social Behavior, 36*(Extra issue), 5-33.

Peterson, P. (1999). How will America pay for the retirement of the baby boom generation? In J. B. Williamson, D. M. Watts-Roy, & E. Kingson (Eds.), *The generational equity debate* (pp. 41-57). New York: Columbia University Press.

Pew Research Center for the People & the Press Survey. (1999, July 13-18). *A few questions about national issues.* Retrieved February 22, 2000, from PollingReport.com on the World Wide Web: pollingreport.com/prioriti.htm

Phillipson, C. (1982). *Capitalism and the construction of old age.* London: Macmillan.

Phillipson, C. (1992). Challenging the "spectre of old age": Community care for older people in the 1990s. In W. Manning & R. Page (Eds.), *Social policy yearbook.* London: Social Policy Association.

Phillipson, C. (1998). *Reconstructing old age: New agendas in social theory and practice.* London: Sage.

Phillipson, C. (1999). The social construction of retirement. In M. Minkler & C. L. Estes (Eds.), *Critical gerontology: Perspectives from political and moral economy* (pp. 315-325). Amityville, NY: Baywood.

Phillipson, C., & Walker, A. (1986). *Ageing and social policy: A critical assessment.* Brookfield, VT: Gower.

Piven, F. F., & Cloward, R. A. (1997). *The breaking of the American social compact.* New York: New Press, Distributed by Norton.

Plotkin, S., & Scheuerman, W. E.. (1994). *Private interest, public spending: Balanced budget conservatism and the fiscal crisis.* Boston, MA: South End.

Porter, A. I. (1995). *The path to poverty: An analysis of women's retirement income* (Mother's Day Report). Washington, DC: Older Women's League.

President's Council on Physical Fitness. (1979). *Physical fitness/sports medicine* (Publication of the President's Council on Physical Fitness and Sports, No. 1). Washington, DC: Government Printing Office.

Preston, S. H., Elo, I. T., Rosenwaike, I., & Hill, M. (1996). African-American mortality at older ages: Results of a matching study. *Demography, 33,* 193-209.

The public market. (1998). *SeniorCare Investor, 10,* 1.

Quadagno, J. (1989). Generational equity and the politics of the welfare state. *Politics & Society, 17*(3), 353-377.

Quadagno, J. (1999a). Creating a capital investment welfare state: The new American exceptionalism? [1998 presidential address] *American Sociologic Review, 64*(1), 1-11.

Quadagno, J. (1999b). Social Security and the myth of the entitlement "crisis." In J. B. Williamson, D. M. Watts-Roy, & E. Kingson (Eds.), *The generational equity debate* (pp. 140-156). New York: Columbia University Press.

Quadagno, J., & Reid, J. (1999). The political economy perspective in aging. In V. L. Bengtson & K. W. Schaie (Eds.), *Handbook of theories of aging* (pp. 344-358). New York: Springer.

Quadagno, J. S. (1988). *The transformation of old age security: Class and politics in the American welfare state.* Chicago: University of Chicago Press.

Quadagno, J. S. (1994). *The color of welfare: How racism undermined the war on poverty.* New York: Oxford University Press.

Rahn, R. W., & Simonson, K. D. (1980). Tax policy for retirement programs. *Retirement income: Who gets how much and who pays?* Washington, DC: Government Research Corporation.

Redclift, N., & Mingione, E. (Eds.). (1985). *Beyond employment: Household, gender, and subsistence.* New York: Basil Blackwell.

Relman, A. S. (1980). The new medical-industrial complex. *New England Journal of Medicine, 303*(17), 963-970.

Relman, A. S. (1986). The medical industrial complex: Where is it taking us? In P. Conrad & R. Kern (Eds.), *The sociology of health and illness: Critical perspectives* (pp. 240-246). New York: St. Martin's.

Renaud, M. (1975). On the structural constraints to state intervention in health. *International Journal of Health Services, 5*(4), 559-571.

Rice, D., & Michel, M. (1998). *Women and Medicare* (Fact sheet). San Francisco: University California, Institute for Health and Aging, for the Henry J. Kaiser Family Foundation and OWL: The Voice of Midlife and Older Women.

Rice, D. P., & Feldman, J. J. (1983). Living longer in the US: Demographic changes in health needs of the elderly. *Milbank Memorial Fund Quarterly/Health and Society, 61*(3), 391.

Rice, T. H. (1998). *The economics of health reconsidered.* Chicago: Health Administration Press.

Riley, M. W. (1998). Successful aging. *The Gerontologist, 38*(2), 151.

Riley, M. W., Foner, A., & Riley, J. W., Jr. (1999). The aging and society paradigm. In V. L. Bengtson & K. W. Schaie (Eds.), *Handbook of theories of aging* (pp. 327-343). New York: Springer.

Riley, M. W., Johnson, M., & Foner, A. (1972). A sociology of age stratification. In M. W. Riley, A. Foner, M. E. Moore, B. Hess, & B. K. Roth (Eds.), *Aging and society* (Vol. 3). New York: Russell Sage.

Riley, M. W., & Riley, J. W. (1994a). Age integration and the lives of older people. *The Gerontologist, 34*(1), 110-115.

Riley, M. W., & Riley, J. W. (1994b). Structural lag: Past and future. In M. W. Riley, R. L. Kahn, & A. Foner (Eds.), *Age and structural lag: Society's failure to provide meaningful opportunities in work, family, and leisure* (pp. 15-36). New York: John Wiley.

Rivlin, A. M., & Wiener, J. M. (1988). *Caring for the disabled elderly: Who will pay?* Washington, DC: Brookings Institution.

Robert, S. A. (1999). Socioeconomic position and health: The independent contribution of community socioeconomic context. *Annual Review of Sociology, 25,* 489-516.

Robert, S. A., & House, J. S. (2000). Socioeconomic inequalities in health: An enduring sociological problem. In C. E. Bird, P. Conrad, & A. M. Fremont (Eds.), *Handbook of medical sociology* (5th ed., pp. 79-97). Upper Saddle River, NJ: Prentice Hall.

Robertson, A. (1990). The politics of Alzheimer's disease: A case study in apocalyptic demography. *International Journal of Health Services, 20*(3), 429-442.

Robertson, A. (1999). Beyond apocalyptic demography: Toward a moral economy of interdependence. In M. Minkler & C. L. Estes (Eds.), *Critical gerontology: Perspectives from political and moral economy* (pp. 75-90). Amityville, NY: Baywood.

Robinson, J. C., & Luft, H. S. (1988). Competition, regulation, and hospital costs, 1982 to 1986 [published erratum appears in JAMA, 1989, *262*(3), 353]. *Journal of the American Medical Association, 260*(18), 2676-2681.

Rodberg, L., & Stevenson, G. (1977). The health care industry in advanced capitalism. *Review of Radical Political Economics, 9,* 104-115.

Rodin, J., & Langer, E. (1977). Long-term effects of a control-relevant intervention with the institutionalized aged. *Journal of Personality and Social Psychology, 35,* 897-902.

Rogot, E. (1992). *A mortality study of 1.3 million persons by demographic, social and economic factors: 1979-1985 follow-up* (Report of the U.S. National Longitudinal Mortality Study). Bethesda, MD: National Institutes of Health, National Heart, Lung, and Blood Institute.

Ronge, V. (1974, March). The politicization of administration in advanced capitalist societies. *Political Studies,* p. 22.

Rose, A. M. (1967). *The power structure: Political process in American society.* London, UK: Oxford University Press.

Roszak, T. (1998). *America the wise: The longevity revolution and the true wealth of nations.* Boston, MA: Houghton Mifflin.

Rowbotham, S. (1981). The trouble with "patriarchy." In F. A. Collective (Ed.), *No turning back: Writings from the women's liberation movement, 1975-80* (pp. 72-78). London: Women's Press.

Rowe, J. W., & Kahn, R. L. (1987). Human aging: Usual and successful. *Science, 237*(4811), 143-149.

Rowe, J. W., & Kahn, R. L. (1997). Successful aging. *The Gerontologist, 37*(4), 433-440.

Rowe, J. W., & Kahn, R. L. (1998). *Successful aging.* New York: Pantheon.

Rubin, G. (1975). The traffic in women. In R. Reiter (Ed.), *Toward an anthropology of women* (pp. 157-210). New York: Monthly Review Press.

Rudney, G. (1987). The scope and dimensions of nonprofit activity. In W. W. Powell (Ed.), *The nonprofit sector: A research handbook* (pp. 55-64). New Haven, CT: Yale University Press.

Ruther, M., & Dobson, A. (1981). Equal treatment and unequal benefits: A reexamination of the use of medical services by race, 1967-1976. *Health Care Financing Review, 2*(3), 55-83.

Salamon, L. (1987a). Of market failure, voluntary failure, and third party government: Toward a theory of government-nonprofit relations in the modern welfare state. In S. A. Ostrander & S. Langton (Eds.), *Shifting the debate: Public/private sector relations in the modern welfare state.* New Brunswick, NJ: Transaction Books.

Salamon, L. (1987b). Partners in public service: The scope and theory of government-nonprofit relations. In W. W. Powell (Ed.), *The nonprofit sector: A research handbook* (pp. 99-117). New Haven, CT: Yale University Press.

Sardar, Z., & Van Loon, B. (1997). *Introducing cultural studies.* New York: Totem.

Sarvasy, W., & Siim, B. (1994). Gender, transitions to democracy, and citizenship. *Social Politics: International Studies in Gender, State & Society, 1*(3), 249-255.

Sassoon, A. S. (1987a). *Gramsci's politics* (2nd ed.). London, UK: Hutchinson.

Sassoon, A. S. (1987b). *Women and the state: The shifting boundaries of public and private.* London: Hutchinson.

Sassoon, A. S. (1991). Equality and difference: The emergence of a new concept of citizenship. In D. McLellan & S. Sayers (Eds.), *Socialism and democracy* (pp. 87-105). Houndmills, Basingstoke, Hampshire, UK: Macmillan.

Scarpaci, J. L. (1989). The theory and practice of health services privatization. In J. L. Scarpaci (Ed.), *Health services privatization in industrial societies* (pp. 1-23). New Brunswick, NJ: Rutgers University Press.

Schaar, J. H. (1984). Legitimacy in the modern state. In W. E. Connolly (Ed.), *Legitimacy and the state* (pp. 104-133). New York: New York University Press.

Schattschneider, E. E. (1960). *The semisovereign people: A realist's view of democracy in America.* New York: Holt, Rinehart & Winston.

Schlesinger, M., Marmor, T. R., & Smithey, R. (1987). Nonprofit and for-profit medical care: Shifting roles and implications for health policy. *Journal of Health Politics, Policy and Law, 12*(3), 427-457.

Scull, A. T. (1977). *Decarceration.* Englewood Cliffs, NJ: Prentice Hall.

Shaughnessy, P. W., Schlenker, R. E., & Hittle, D. F. (1994). Home health care outcomes under capitated and fee-for-service payment. *Health Care Financing Review, 16*(1), 187-222.

Siegel, J. S., & Taeuber, C. M. (1986). Demographic perspectives on the long-lived society. *Daedalus, 115*(1), 77-117.

Sirrocco, A. (1994). *Nursing homes and board and care homes: Data from the 1991 national health provider inventory.* Hyattsville, MD: U.S. Department of Health and Human Services, Public Health Service, Centers for Disease Control and Prevention, National Center for Health Statistics.

Skinner, J., & Fisher, E. (1997). Regional disparities in Medicare expenditures: An opportunity for reform. *National Tax Journal, 50*(3), 413-425.

Skocpol, T. (1992). *Protecting soldiers and mothers: The political origins of social policy in the United States.* Cambridge, MA: Belknap Press of Harvard University Press.

Slaughter, J. (1997, November). Doctors unite: Corporate medicine and the surprising trend of doctor unionization. *Multinational Monitor,* pp. 22-24.

Smeeding, T., Estes, C. L., & Glasse, L. (1999). *Social Security reform and older women: Improving the system* (Report for the Task Force on Women). Washington, DC: Gerontological Society of America.

Smith, D. (1990). *The conceptual practices of power: A feminist sociology of knowledge.* Boston, MA: Northeastern University Press.

Smith, S., Freeland, M., Heffler, S., McKusick, D., & the Health Expenditures Projection Team. (1998). The next ten years of health spending: What does the future hold? *Health Affairs, 17*(5), 128-140.

Social Security Administration. (1998a). *Fast facts & figures about Social Security* (Fact sheet). Washington, DC: Social Security Administration, Office of Research, Evaluation and Statistics.

Social Security Administration. (1998b). *Income of the population 55 or older.* Washington, DC: Social Security Administration.

Soldo, B. J., Agree, E. M., & Wolf, D. A. (1989). The balance between formal and informal care. In M. G. Ory & K. Bonds (Eds.), *Aging and health care: Social science and policy perspectives* (pp. 193-216). London: Routledge.

Soldo, B. J., & Manton, K. G. (1985). Health status and service needs of the oldest old: Current patterns and future trends. *Milbank Memorial Fund Quarterly/Health and Society, 63*(2), 286-319.

Southwick, K. (1990). More merger mania among drugmakers. *Healthweek, 4*(1), 51.

Srinivasan, S., Levitt, L., & Lundy, J. (1998). Wall Street's love affair with health care. *Health Affairs, 17*(4), 126-131.

Starr, P. (1982). *The social transformation of American medicine.* New York: Basic Books.

Stefancic, J., & Delgado, R. (1996). *No mercy: How conservative think tanks and foundations changed America's social agenda.* Philadelphia, PA: Temple University Press.

Steinberg, R. (1988, June 28-29). *Testimony of Richard Steinberg.* Paper presented at the Hearing on Nonprofit Competition, Committee on Small Business, House of Representatives, 100th Cong. 2d Sess., Washington, DC.

Steuerle, E. (1999). *The treatment of the family and divorce in the Social Security program* (Report). Washington, DC: U.S. Senate Special Committee on Aging.

Stevens, R. (1982). "A poor sort of memory": Voluntary hospitals and government before the depression. *Milbank Memorial Fund Quarterly/Health and Society, 60*(4), 551-584.

Stevens, R. (1983). Comparisons in health care: Britain as a contrast to the U.S. In D. Mechanic (Ed.), *Handbook of health, health care, and the health professions* (pp. 281-304). New York: Free Press.

Stone, A., & Harpham, E. J. (1982). *The political economy of public policy.* Beverly Hills, CA: Sage.

Stone, R., Cafferata, G., & Sangl, J. (1987). Caregivers of the frail elderly: A national profile. *The Gerontologist, 27*, 616-627.

Strauss, A. L., & Corbin, J. M. (1988). *Shaping a new health care system: The explosion of chronic illness as a catalyst for change.* San Francisco: Jossey-Bass.

Street, D., & Quadagno, J. (1993). The state, the elderly, and the intergenerational contract: Toward a new political economy of aging. In K. Schaie & A. Achenbaum (Eds.), *Societal Impact on Aging* (pp. 130-150). New York: Springer.

Swain, F. (1988, June 28-29). *Testimony of Frank S. Swain.* Paper presented at the Hearing on Nonprofit Competition, Committee on Small Business, House of Representatives, 100th Cong. 2d Sess., Washington, DC.

Syme, S. L., & Berkman, L. F. (1976, July). Social class, susceptibility, and sickness. *American Journal of Epidemiology,* pp. 1-8.

Szasz, A. (1990). The labor impacts of policy changes in health care: How federal policy transformed home health organizations and their labor practices. *Journal of Health Politics, Policy, and Law, 1,* 191-210.

Tabb, W. K. (1999). Labor and the imperialism of finance. *Monthly Review: An Independent Socialist Magazine, 51*(5), 1-13.

Taeuber, C. M. (1992). *Sixty-five plus in America* (Report). Washington, DC: U.S. Bureau of the Census.

Tarabusi, C. C., & Vickery, G. (1998). Globalization of the pharmaceutical industry, Parts I and II. *International Journal of Health Services, 28,* 67-105, 281-303.

Taylor, D. (Ed.). (1996). *Critical social policy, a reader: Social policy and social relations.* London, UK; Thousand Oaks, CA: Sage.

Taylor, R. J., & Chatters, L. M. (1991). Extended family networks of older black adults. *Journal of Gerontology, 46,* S210-S217.

Therborn, G. (1978). *What does the ruling class do when it rules? State apparatuses and state power under feudalism, capitalism and socialism.* Thetford, Norfolk, UK: Lowe & Brydore.

Therborn, G. (1980). *The ideology of power and the power of ideology.* New York: NLB, dist. in the U.S. by Schocken Books.

Thompson, E. P. (1963). *The making of the English working class.* New York: Vintage.

Thompson, K. (1986). *Beliefs and ideology.* New York: Tavistock.

Thurow, L. C. (1999). Generational equity and the birth of a revolutionary class. In J. B. Williamson, D. M. Watts-Roy, & E. Kingson (Eds.), *The generational equity debate* (pp. 58-74). New York: Columbia University Press.

Townsend, P. (1981). The structured dependency of the elderly: A creation of social policy in the twentieth century. *Ageing and Society, 1*(1), 5-28.

Tres, J. (1995). Older Americans in the 1990s and beyond. *Population Bulletin, 50*(2).

Turner, B. (1999). *Classical sociology.* London, UK: Sage.

Tussing, A. (1971). A dual welfare system. In I. L. Horowitz & C. Levey (Eds.), *Social realities.* New York: Harper & Row.

Twine, F. (1994). *Citizenship and social rights: The interdependence of self and society.* London, UK; Thousand Oaks, CA: Sage.

Ubel, P. A., DeKay, M. L., Baron, J., & Asch, D. A. (1996). Cost effectiveness analysis in a setting of budget constraints: Is it equitable? *New England Journal of Medicine, 334*(18), 1174-1177.

Ulbrich, P. M., & Bradsher, J. E. (1993). Perceived support, help seeking, and adjustment to stress among older black and white women living alone. *Journal of Aging and Health, 5,* 365-386.

U.S. Bureau of the Census. (1993). *1990 Census of the population and housing series CPH-L-74, modified and actual age, sex, race, and Hispanic origin; 2050 from population projections of the United States by age, race, and Hispanic origin: 1993-2050*

(Current population reports Series P25-1104). Washington, DC: Government Printing Office.

U.S. Bureau of the Census. (1994). *Marital status and living arrangements: March 1993* (Current population reports). Washington, DC: Government Printing Office.

U.S. Bureau of the Census. (1996). *65+ in the United States* (Current population reports special studies). Washington, DC: Author.

U.S. Bureau of the Census. (2000). *Projections of the total resident population by 5-year age groups, race, and Hispanic origin with special age categories: Middle Series, 2050 to 2070.* Washington, DC: Author. Retrieved September 19, 2000, from the World Wide Web: www.census.gov/population/projections/nation/summary/np-t3-g.txt

U.S. Department of Commerce. (1990). *Health and medical services* (U.S. Industrial Outlook 1990). Washington, DC: International Trade Administration.

U.S. Department of Health, Education and Welfare. (1979). *Healthy people* (Surgeon General's Report on Health Promotion and Disease Prevention). Washington, DC: Public Health Service.

U.S. Department of Health and Human Services. (1989). *Health United States, 1989* (DHHS Publication No. 90-1232). Hyattsville, MD: Author.

U.S. Department of Health and Human Services. (1997). *Home health agencies* (unpublished data). Baltimore, MD: Health Care Financing Administration.

U.S. Department of Health and Human Services. (1998). *Healthy people 2010* (Surgeon General's Report on Health Promotion and Disease Prevention). Washington, DC: Public Health Service.

U.S. Department of Health and Human Services. (1999). *Health, United States, 1999: Health and aging chartbook* (DHHS Publication No. PHS 99-1232-1). Hyattsville, MD: Author.

Van Til, J. (1982). Volunteering and democratic theory. In J. D. Harman (Ed.), *Volunteerism in the eighties: Fundamental issues in voluntary action* (pp. 199-220). Washington, DC: University Press of America.

Van Til, J. (1987). The three sectors: Voluntarism in a changing political economy. In S. A. Ostrander & S. Langton (Eds.), *Shifting the debate: Public/private sector relations in the modern welfare state* (pp. 50-63). New Brunswick, NJ: Transaction Books.

Vaughan, G. (1997). *For-giving: A feminist criticism of exchange.* Austin, TX: Plain View Press.

Verbrugge, L. M. (1989). The dynamics of population aging and health. In S. J. Lewis (Ed.), *Aging and health: Linking research and public policy* (pp. 23-40). Chelsea, MI: Lewis.

Vladeck, B. C. (1980). *Unloving care: The nursing home tragedy.* New York: Basic Books.

Waitzkin, H. (1983). *The second sickness: Contradictions of capitalist health care.* New York: Free Press/Macmillan.

Waitzkin, H. (1989). Social structures of medical oppression: A Marxist view. In P. Brown, (Ed.), *Perspectives in medical sociology* (pp. 166-178). Belmont, CA: Wadsworth.

Waitzman, N. J. (1988). *The occupational determinants of health: A labor market segmentation analysis.* Unpublished doctoral dissertation, American University, Washington, DC.

Walby, S. (1986). *Patriarchy at work: Patriarchal and capitalist relations in employment.* Minneapolis: University of Minnesota Press.

Waldo, D. R., Sonnefeld, S. T., McKusick, D. R., & Arnett, R. H. D. (1989). Health expenditures by age group, 1977 and 1987. *Health Care Financing Review, 10*(4), 111-120.

Walker, A. (1980). Social creation of poverty and dependency in old age. *Journal of Social Policy, 9*(1), 49-75.

Walker, A. (1981). Towards a political economy of old age. *Ageing and Society, 1*(1), 73-94.

Walker, A. (1984). *Social planning: A strategy for social welfare.* Oxford, UK: Basil Blackwell.

Walker, A. (1991). *Intergenerational relations and welfare restructuring: The social construction of a generational problem.* Paper presented at the Conference on the New Contract Between the Generations: Social Science Perspectives on Cohorts in the 21st Century, USC, Los Angeles, CA.

Walker, A. (1999). Public policy and theories of aging: Constructing and reconstructing old age. In V. L. Bengston & K. W. Schaie (Eds.), *Handbook of theories of aging* (pp. 361-378). New York: Springer.

Wallace, S. P. (2000). American health promotion: Where individualism rules. *The Gerontologist, 40*(3), 373-377.

Wallace, S. P., Cohen, J., Schnelle, J., Kane, R. L., & Ouslander, J. G. (2000). Managed care and multi-level long-term care providers: Reluctant partners. *The Gerontologist, 40*(2), 197-205.

Wallace, S. P., Enriquez-Haass, V., & Markides, K. (1998). The consequences of color-blind health policy for older racial and ethnic minorities. *Stanford Law Review, 9*(2), 329-346.

Weber, M. (1946). Class, status and party. In H. H. Gerth & C. W. Mills (Eds.), *From Max Weber: Essays in sociology* (pp. 180-195). New York: Oxford University Press.

Weisbrod, B. A. (1998). *To profit or not to profit: The commercial transformation of the nonprofit sector.* Cambridge, UK: Cambridge University Press.

Wennberg, J. E., & Cooper, M. (1997). Variability in Medicare spending by region. In J. E. Wennberg & M. Cooper (Eds.), *Dartmouth atlas of health care: 1998.* Chicago: American Hospital Publications

White House Conference on Aging, 1981 (final report). Washington, DC: U.S. Department of Health, Education and Welfare.

Wilkinson, R. (Ed.). (1986). *Class and health: Research and longitudinal data.* London: Tavistock.

Williams, D. R. (1990). Socioeconomic differentials in health: A review and redirection. *Social Psychology Quarterly, 53*, 81-99.

Williams, D. R., & Collins, C. (1995). U.S. socioeconomic and racial differences in health: Patterns and explanations. *Annual Review of Sociology, 21*, 349-396.

Williams, F. (1996). Racism and the discipline of social policy: A critique of welfare theory. In D. Taylor (Ed.), *Critical social policy: A reader* (pp. 48-78). Thousand Oaks, CA: Sage.

Williamson, J. B., Watts-Roy, D. M., & Kingson, E. (Eds.). (1999). *The generational equity debate.* New York: Columbia University Press.

Wing, S., Manton, K. G., Stallard, E., Hames, C. G., & Tryoler, H. A. (1985). The black/white mortality crossover: Investigation in a community-based study. *Journal of Gerontology, 40*, 78-84.

Wohl, S. (1984). *The medical industrial complex.* New York: Harmony Books.

Wolf, D. A. (1999). The family as provider of long-term care: Efficiency, equity, and externalities. *Journal of Aging and Studies, 11,* 360-382.

Wood, J. B. (1991). Caregivers as controllers: Women and long-term care and cost-containment. *Journal of Aging and Social Policy, 3,* 31-46.

Wood, J. B., & Estes, C. L. (1986). Health care cost containment and nonprofit homemaker/chore agencies. *Caring, 5*(9), 26-34.

Wood, J. B., & Estes, C. L. (1988). "Medicalization" of community services for the elderly. *Health and Social Work, 13*(1), 35-42.

Wood, J. B., & Estes, C. L. (1990). The impact of DRGs on community-based service providers: Implications for the elderly. *American Journal of Public Health, 80*(7), 840-843.

Wood, J. B., Hughes, R. G., & Estes, C. L. (1986). Community health centers and the elderly: A potential new alliance. *Journal of Community Health, 11*(2), 137-146.

Woolhandler, S., & Himmelstein, D. (1999). When money is the mission: The high costs of investor-owned care. *New England Journal of Medicine, 341*(6), 444-446.

Wright, E. O. (1989). *The debate on classes.* New York: Verso.

Wright, E. O. (1997). *Class counts: Comparative studies in class analysis.* New York: Cambridge University Press.

Yen, I. H., & Kaplan, G. A. (1999). Neighborhood social environment and risk of death: Multilevel evidence from the Alameda County Study. *American Journal of Epidemiology, 149*(10), 898-907.

Yen, I. H., & Syme, S. L. (1999). The social environment and health: A discussion of the epidemiologic literature. *Annual Review of Public Health, 20,* 287-308.

Young, D. (1988, June 28-29). *Testimony of Dennis R., Young.* Paper presented at the Hearing on Nonprofit Competition, Committee on Small Business, House of Representatives, 100th Cong. 2d Sess., Washington, DC.

Zola, I. K. (1975). In the name of health and illness: On some socio-political consequences of medical influence. *Social Science and Medicine, 9*(2), 83-87.

Zuckerman, D. (1999, May/June). The derailing of Social Security. *Extra!* pp. 13-14.

Index

About the Authors

Carroll L. Estes, Ph.D., is Professor of Sociology at the University of California, San Francisco (UCSF). She is the founding and former Director of the Institute for Health & Aging (1979-1998) and the former Chair of the Department of Social and Behavioral Sciences, School of Nursing, UCSF. She is a member of the Institute of Medicine, the National Academy of Sciences, and past President of the Gerontological Society of America, the American Society on Aging, and the Association for Gerontology in Higher Education. She has served as consultant to the U.S. Commissioner of Social Security and to U.S. Senate and House committees for more than two decades. Her work is nationally and internationally recognized, and her book, *The Aging Enterprise,* is considered one of the classic texts in the field of aging research.

Associates

Robert R. Alford, Ph.D., is Distinguished Professor of Sociology at the City University of New York Graduate Center. He is the author of books on comparative voting behavior, urban political cultures, health care politics, theories of the state, and, most recently, *The Craft of Inquiry* (1998). He is currently working on a project on the production of political culture—specifically, the emergence of symbolic icons in the course of public investigations.

Elizabeth A. Binney was a doctoral student in the Department of Social Behavioral Sciences and Research Associate for the Institute for Health & Aging, University of California, San Francisco. A former National Institute on Aging

283

Predoctoral Fellow, she conducted research on the political economy of aging and health policy and older women's issues, including the social construction and political economy of osteoporosis.

Julia E. Bradsher, Ph.D., is a health services researcher with Abt Associates, Inc., in Cambridge, Massachusetts. Her work includes evaluation and policy research on Medicare, insurance for the uninsured, and organizational and financial arrangements in managed care. Prior to her work with Abt Associates, she was a senior research scientist at the New England Research Institutes where she directed the Coordinating Center for the Study of Women's Health Across the Nation.

Liz Close, R.N., Ph.D., is Professor and Chair, Department of Nursing, School of Natural Sciences, Sonoma State University, Rohnert Park, California. She was awarded a National Institute of Aging predoctoral fellowship in socio-cultural gerontology during graduate studies at the University of California, San Francisco, where she earned her doctorate in sociology. Her research focuses on the structural intersection of paid and unpaid labor in the provision of home health care.

Chiquita A. Collins, Ph.D., is a postdoctoral fellow with the Robert Wood Johnson Foundation Scholars in Health Policy Research Program at the University of California, Berkeley. She is also Assistant Professor at the University of Illinois at Chicago in the Departments of Sociology and African-American Studies. Her areas of interest include racial and socioeconomic differentials in health, racism and health, social epidemiology, and social demography.

Anne Hays Egan is an organizational development, planning, and evaluation consultant. Part of her work in applied research and consultation addresses the impact of devolution on nonprofit agencies and community systems as well as strategies needed to respond. She has authored and published *The Digest of Nonprofit Management* (1988-1992), *Medicaid and Block Grant Primer* (1995), and *The Devolution Toolkit* (1996, revised 1998).

Charlene Harrington, Ph.D., is Professor of Sociology and Nursing in the Department of Social and Behavioral Sciences, School of Nursing, University of California, San Francisco. She was elected to the Institute of Medicine and is a Fellow in the American Academy of Nursing. Her major interest is in nursing home quality and regulation. She served on the Institute of Medicine (IOM) Committee on Nursing Home Regulation, whose 1986 report led to the passage of the Nursing Home Reform Act of 1987. She recently developed a Nursing Home Consumer Information System and currently serves on an IOM committee to study quality in long-term care.

Karen W. Linkins, Ph.D., is Senior Manager at The Lewin Group, where she is conducting several studies on state variations in home- and community-based waivers, including an evaluation of the family care program in Wisconsin. She is also leading evaluations of state-based implementation of assertive community treatment programs and the effectiveness of pre-admission screening for nursing home residents. Her other research interests include the political economy of long-term care and pharmaceuticals, and mental health and substance abuse service access for the elderly.

Marty Lynch, Ph.D., is Executive Director of the Over 60 Health Center in Berkeley, California, and a lecturer at the Institute for Health & Aging, University of California, San Francisco (UCSF). He was one of 10 recipients of a Robert Wood Johnson Community Health Leadership Award in 1995. His research has been in the areas of long-term care reform, medical services in social/health maintenance organizations, and managed care for the elderly.

Jane L. Mahakian, Ph.D., is Principal of Pacific Senior Services, a West Coast geriatric care management company that specializes in assisting older adults who suffer from memory loss, and their families. She is Visiting Adjunct Professor at the Institute for Health & Aging, University of California, San Francisco (UCSF), and past Director of the UCSF Elder Care Referral Program. She also serves as consultant to assisted-living facilities and conducts corporate seminars and training on elder care, work/life issues, and healthy and productive aging.

David N. Pellow, Ph.D., is Assistant Professor of Ethnic Studies and Sociology at the University of Colorado at Boulder. His research and teaching focus on social movements, environmental justice, and the sociology of work and health. He is coauthor (with Adam Weinberg and Allan Schnaiberg) of *Urban Recycling and the Search for Sustainable Community Development.*

Steven P. Wallace, Ph.D., is Associate Professor at the School of Public Health, University of California, Los Angeles (UCLA), and Associate Director of the UCLA Center for Health Policy Research. In 2000, he was a Fulbright Scholar in Chile, where he conducted research and lectured on health policy for older persons in Latin America. His other research focuses on the impact of race and ethnicity on the use of long-term care in the United States and the consequences of public policies for the health and quality of life of racial and ethnic minority elderly.

Tracy A. Weitz, M.P.A., is Project Director for the Center for Reproductive Health Research and Policy at the University of California, San Francisco (UCSF). She is also the former Evaluation Director and a current senior adviser for the UCSF National Center of Excellence in Women's Health. Her current research interests include ongoing work on the rhetorical implications of public abortion discourse, the ostracism of child-free women from the women's health movement, and the merging of younger and older women's health.